Assessment

an

Incredibly Easy!®

Pocket
Guide

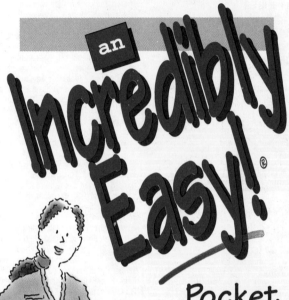

LIPPINCOTT WILLIAMS & WILKINS
A **Wolters Kluwer** Company

Philadelphia • Baltimore • New York • London
Buenos Aires • Hong Kong • Sydney • Tokyo

Staff

Executive Publisher
Judith A. Schilling McCann, RN, MSN

Editorial Director
David Moreau

Clinical Director
Joan M. Robinson, RN, MSN

Senior Art Director
Arlene Putterman

Art Director
Mary Ludwicki

Editorial Project Manager
Jaime Stockslager Buss

Clinical Project Manager
Collette Bishop Hendler, RN, BS, CCRN

Editors
Rita Breedlove, Liz Schaeffer,
Beth Wegerbauer

Copy Editors
Kimberly Bilotta (supervisor), Scotti Cohn,
Shana Harrington, Kelly Pavlovsky,
Pamela Wingrod

Designer
Lynn Foulk

Illustrator
Bot Roda

Digital Composition Services
Diane Paluba (manager), Joyce Rossi Biletz

Manufacturing
Patricia K. Dorshaw (director),
Beth J. Welsh

Editorial Assistants
Megan L. Aldinger, Karen J. Kirk,
Linda K. Ruhf

Indexer
Barbara Hodgson

ASSMTIEPG010705 — D N O S A J
07 06 05   10 9 8 7 6 5 4 3

Library of Congress Cataloging-in-Publication
Assessment : an incredibly easy pocket guide
    p. ; cm.
    Includes bibliographical references and
    1. Nursing assessment — Handbooks, m
      etc. I. Lippincott Williams & Wilkins.
    [DNLM: 1. Nursing Assessment — meth
    Handbooks. WY 49 A8456 2006]
RT48.A8733 2006
616.07'5--dc22
ISBN 1-58255-431-5 (alk. paper)   200

ntents

Contributors and consultants

Deborah A. Andris, RN,CS, MSN, APNP
Nurse Practitioner
Bariatric Surgery Program
Medical College of Wisconsin
Milwaukee

Jemma Bailey-Kunte, APRN-BC, MS, FNP
Clinical Lecturer
Binghamton (N.Y.) University
Nurse Practitioner
Lourdes Hospital
Binghamton

Cheryl A. Bean, APRN,BC, DSN, ANP, AOCN
Associate Professor
Indiana University School of Nursing
Indianapolis

Natalie Burkhalter, RN, MSN, ACNP, CS, FNP
Associate Professor
Texas A&M International University
Laredo

Shelba Durston, RN, MSN, CCRN
Nursing Instructor
San Joaquin Delta College
Stockton, Calif.
Staff Nurse
San Joaquin General Hospital
French Camp, Calif.

Tamara D. Espejo, RN, MS
Registered Nurse and Clinical Educator
Aurora Behavioral Healthcare-Charter Oak
Covina, Calif.

Michelle L. Foley, RN,C, MA
Director of Nursing Education
Charles E. Gregory School of Nursing
Raritan Bay Medical Center
Perth Amboy, N.J.

Catherine B. Holland, RN, PhD, APRN,BC ANP, CNS
Associate Professor
Southeastern Louisiana University
Baton Rouge

Julia Anne Isen, RN, MS, FNP-C
Nurse Practitioner — Internal Medicin
Veteran Administration Medical Cente
San Francisco
Assistant Clinical Professor
School of Nursing
University of California at San Francisc

Nancy Banfield Johnson, RN, MSN, AN (inactive)
Nurse-manager
Kendal at Ithaca (N.Y.)

Gary R. Jones, MSN, CNS, FNP
ARNP, Disease Management Program
Mercy Health Center
Fort Scott, Kans.

Vanessa C. Kramasz, RN, MSN, FNP-C
Nursing Faculty & Family Nurse Practi
Gateway Technical College
Kenosha, Wis.

Priscilla A. Lee, MN, FNP
Instructor in Nursing
Moorpark (Calif.) College

Susan Luck, RN, MS, CCN
Director of Nutrition
Biodoron Immunology Center
Hollywood, Fla.

Ann S. McQueen, RNC, MSN, CRNP
Family Nurse Practitioner
Healthlink Medical Center
Southampton, Pa.

O'Donnell, RN, BSN
nistrator Community Surgery Center
nunity Hospital
ter, Ind.

am J. Pawlyshyn, RN, MS, MN, APRN,BC
e Practitioner Consultant
England Geriatrics
Springfield, Mass.

rine Pence, RN, MSN, CCRN
tant Professor
Samaritan College of Nursing
nnati

Plambeck, RN, BSN
endent Consultant
aukee, Wis.

sa Pulvano, RN, BSN
ng Educator
n County Vocational Technical School
urst, N.J.

ca Narvaez Ramirez, RN, MSN
ty
rsity of the Incarnate Word
ntonio, Tex.

a Reed, MSN, FNP
iate Professor
ington State Community College
etta, Ohio

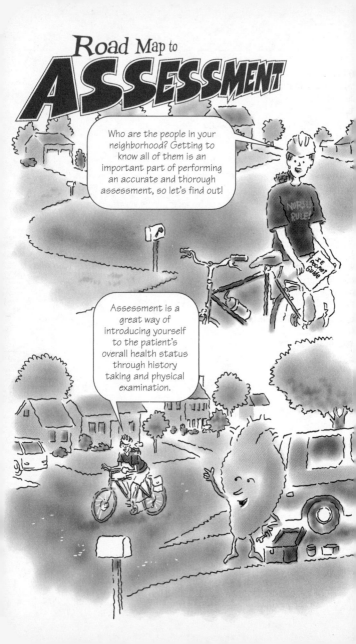

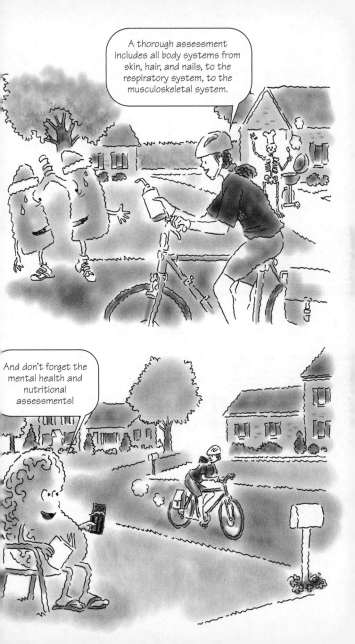

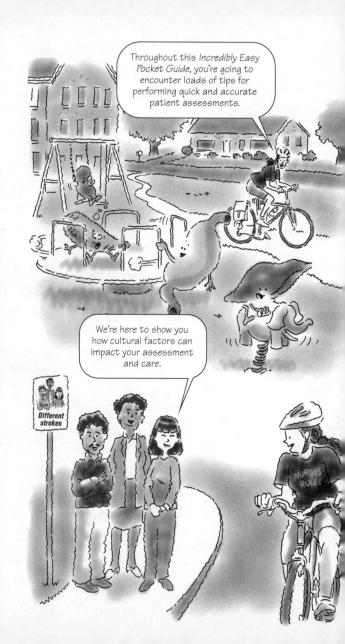

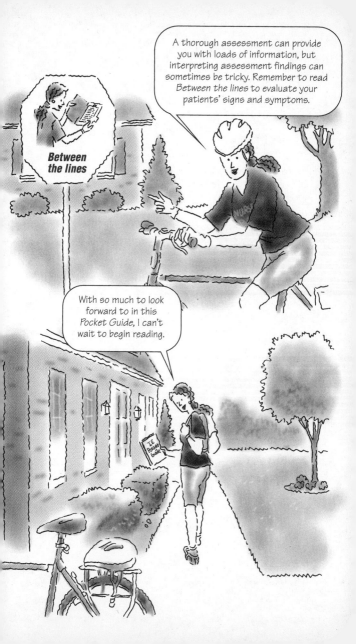

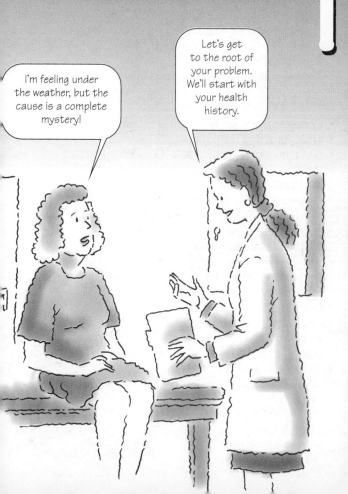

Health history overview

- Helps you uncover significant problems and make an appropriate care plan
- Involves collecting two kinds of data
  - *Objective data* — obtained through observation (red, swollen arm) and verifiable (patient complains of arm pain)
  - *Subjective data* — gathered solely from the patient's own account ("my head hurts") and can't be verified by anyone other than the patient
- Explores past and present problems

Beginning the interview

- Choose a quiet, private, well-lit interview setting.
- Make sure that the patient is comfortable.
- Sit facing the patient, 3′ to 4′ (1 to 1.5 m) away.
- Introduce yourself and explain the purpose of the health history and assessment.
- Establish a rapport with the patient, and explain what you'll cover during the interview.
- Assure the patient that everything he says will be kept confidential.
- Tell the patient how long the interview will last, and ask him what he hopes to gain from the health assessment.
- Use touch sparingly because many people aren't comfortable with strangers touching them.
- Assess the patient to see whether language barriers exist.
  - Does he speak and understand English?
  - Can he hear you?

The health history explores the patient's past and present problems.

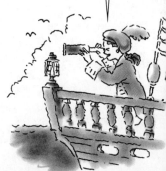

Different strokes

Overcoming interviewing obstacles

Lost in translation?

Your facility may have interpreters you can call on for help if a patient doesn't speak English. A trained medical interpreter — one who's familiar with medical terminology, interpreting techniques, and patient's rights — would be ideal.

Tell the interpreter to translate the patient's words verbatim.

Avoid using one of the patient's family members or friends as an interpreter. Doing so would violate the patient's right to confidentiality.

Breaking the sound barrier

If a patient is hearing impaired, make sure the light is bright enough for him to see your lips move.

Face the patient and speak slowly and clearly.

If needed, have the patient use an assistive device, such as a hearing aid or an amplifier.

If your facility has a sign-language interpreter and the patient uses sign language, request assistance.

Speak slowly and clearly, using easy-to-understand language.

Avoid using medical terms and jargon.

Address the patient by his formal name.

- Don't call him by his first name unless he asks you to.

- Show respect for the patient, which encourages him to trust you and provide accurate and complete information.

Nonverbal communication strategies

Listen attentively and make eye contact frequently.

Use reassuring gestures.

- Nod your head to encourage the patient to keep talking.

Different strokes

Overcoming cultural barriers

To maintain a good relationship with your patient, remember that his cultural behaviors and beliefs may differ from your own. For example, most people in the United States make eye contact when talking with others. In contrast, people from several other cultures — including Native Americans, Asians, and people from Arabic-speaking countries — may find eye contact disrespectful or aggressive.

- Watch for nonverbal clues that indicate the patient is uncomfortable or unsure about how to answer a question. For example, he might:
  - lower his voice
  - glance around uneasily.
- Be aware that your nonverbal behavior might cause the patient to stop talking or become defensive. You might appear
  - closed off from him if you cross your arms
  - bored or rushed if you glance at your watch.
- Observe the patient closely to see whether he understands each question.
- If he doesn't seem to understand, repeat questions using different words or appropriate examples.

Verbal communication strategies

- *Open-ended questions* let the patient respond freely. Examples include:
  - How did you fall?
  - How do you feel?
- *Closed questions* elicit one- or two-word responses, such as "yes" or "not today." Examples include:
  - Do you ever have pain in your chest?
  - Do you live alone?

Moments of *silence* during the interview encourage the patient to continue talking and allow you to assess his ability to organize his thoughts.

Facilitation encourages the patient to continue with his story. For example:
- Say, "Please continue."
- Say, "Go on."

Confirmation ensures that you and the patient are on the same track. For example:
- Say, "If I understand you correctly, you said…" and then repeat the information the patient gave.

Two ways to ask

Open-ended questions
- Require the patient to express feelings, opinions, and ideas.
- Help you gather more information than closed questions.
- Facilitate nurse-patient rapport because they show that you're interested in what the patient has to say.
- Examples include:
  – What caused you to come to the hospital tonight?
  – How would you describe the problems you're having with your breathing?
  – What lung problems, if any, do other members of your family have?

Closed questions
- Elicit answers of one to two words, such as "yes" or "not today."
- Help you "zoom in" on specific points but don't provide the patient an opportunity to elaborate.
- Limit the development of nurse-patient rapport.
- Examples include:
  – Do you ever get short of breath?
  – Are you the only one in your family with lung problems?

- *Reflection* (restating something the patient has just said) helps you obtain more specific information. For example, you can turn a statement into a question:
  – You know you have an ulcer?
  – You know you've had a heart attack?
- Use *clarification* when information is vague or confusing.
  – Say, "What do you mean by…" and then repeat the information.
- *Summarization* (briefly restating what the patient told you) ensures that the data you've collected are accurate and complete. It also lets the patient know that the interview is about to end.
- *Signaling* lets the patient know that you're ready to conclude the interview.
  – I think I have all of the information I need.
  – Is there anything else you would like to add?

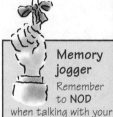

Memory jogger

Remember to **NOD** when talking with your patient:

N: Use **N**onverbal communication.

O: Ask **O**pen-ended questions.

D: **D**on't use terms of endearment, such as "dear" or "darling."

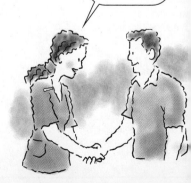

Is there anything else that you think I should know?

eviewing general health

omplete health history requires information from each of
following categories, obtained in this order:

Biographic data
- Name
- Address
- Telephone number
- Birth date
- Age
- Marital status
- Religion and congregation
- Nationality
- Name and telephone number of an emergency contact person
- Primary doctor and other health care providers
- Advance directive

Chief complaint (the patient's reason for seeking care docu-
mented in his exact words)
- How and when did the symptoms develop?
- What led you to seek medical attention?
- How has the problem affected your life and ability to function?

Advance directives

Written documents that state a patient's wishes regarding health
are in the event he becomes unable to make decisions
Allowed by the Patient Self-Determination Act
Health care facilities required to provide information about them
May include:
– name of the person authorized by the patient to make medical decisions if the patient can no longer do so
– specific medical treatment the patient wants or doesn't want, even
if it may hasten his death
– information the patient wants to relay to his loved ones
– name of the patient's primary health care provider
– any other wishes

- Medical history
  - Have you ever been hospitalized? If so, when and why?
  - What childhood illnesses did you have?
  - Are you being treated for any problem? If so, what is it and who's your doctor?
  - Have you ever had surgery? If so, when and why?
  - Are you allergic to anything in the environment or to any drugs or foods? If so, what kind of reaction do you have?
  - Are you taking medications, including over-the-counter preparations, such as aspirin or cough syrup? If so, how much do you take and how often?
  - Do you use home remedies such as homemade ointments?
  - Do you use herbal preparations or take dietary supplements?
  - Do you use other alternative or complementary therapies, such as acupuncture, massage, or chiropractic treatment?
- Family history (can reveal a risk of certain illnesses)
  - Are your mother, father, and siblings alive? If not, how old were they when they died? What caused their deaths?
  - If they're alive, do they have diabetes, high blood pressure, heart disease, asthma, cancer, glaucoma, or other illnesses?
- Psychosocial history (helps determine how the patient feels about himself, his place in society, and his relationships)
  - How have you coped with past medical or emotional crises?
  - Has your life changed recently?
  - Have you noticed any changes in your personality or behavior?
  - How close do you live to health care facilities?
  - Can you get to a health care facility easily?
  - Do you have health insurance?
  - Are you on a fixed income?

Activities of daily living

Find out what's normal for the patient by asking him to describe his typical day. Make sure you cover the following topics.

Diet

- Ask about appetite, special diets, and food allergies.

sking about abuse

Ask two open-ended questions:
– When do you feel safe at home?
– When don't you feel safe?
Watch the patient's reaction:
– Is the patient defensive, hostile, confused, or frightened?
– Does she seem withdrawn?
– Does she show other inappropriate behavior?
If the patient tells you about any type of abuse, you're obligated to
port it. Inform the patient that you must report the incident to local
thorities.

sk who does the cooking and shopping at his house.

ercise and sleep

sk the patient whether he exercises regularly. If so, ask him
describe his exercise program.
sk how many hours the patient sleeps at night, what his
eep pattern is, and whether he feels rested after sleep.
sk him whether he has difficulty sleeping or sleeps too much.

rk and leisure

sk the patient what he does for a living.
sk about hobbies and how he spends his leisure time.

e of tobacco, alcohol, and other drugs

sk the patient whether he smokes cigarettes. If so, ask how
any he smokes each day.
sk whether he drinks alcohol. If so, ask how much he drinks
ach day.
sk whether he uses illicit drugs, such as marijuana and co-
aine. If so, ask how often.

igious observances

sk the patient whether he has religious beliefs that affect his
et, dress, or health practices.

Reviewing structures and systems

Start at the top of the head and work your way down the bo
Ask the patient the following questions.

Head

- Do you get headaches? If so, what triggers them, how often
they occur, how long do they last, and how do you relieve the
- Have you ever had a head injury?

Eyes

- When was your last eye examination?
- Do you wear glasses or contacts?
- Do you have glaucoma, cataracts, or color blindness?
- Does light bother your eyes?
- Do you have excessive tearing or blurred or double vision?

Ears

- Do you have loss of balance, ringing in your ears, deafness,
poor hearing?
- Have you ever had ear surgery? If so, why and when?
- Do you wear a hearing aid?
- Do you have pain, swelling, or discharge from your ears?

Nose

- Have you ever had nasal surgery? If so, why and when?
- Have you ever had a sinus infection or nosebleeds?
- Do you have nasal problems that impair your ability to sme
- Do nasal problems cause breathing difficulties, frequent
sneezing, or discharge?

Mouth and throat

- Do you have mouth sores, a dry mouth, loss of taste, a
toothache, or bleeding gums?
- Do you wear dentures?
- Do you have a sore throat, fever, or chills?

Do you often have a sore throat? If so, have you seen a doctor for this?

Do you have difficulty swallowing ? If so, is the problem with solids or liquids? What, if anything, makes it go away?

Neck

Do you have swelling, soreness, lack of movement, stiffness, or pain in your neck? How long have you had this symptom? Does anything relieve it or aggravate it?

Respiratory system

Do you have shortness of breath on exertion or while lying down?

How many pillows do you use at night?

Does breathing cause pain or wheezing?

Do you have a productive cough? If so, do you cough up blood?

Do you have night sweats?

Have you ever had pneumonia, asthma, or emphysema?

Do you have frequent respiratory tract infections?

Have you ever had a chest X-ray or tuberculin skin test? If so, when and what were the results?

Cardiovascular system

Do you have shortness of breath, a persistent cough, chest pain, palpitations, irregular heartbeat, or fast heartbeat?

Have you ever had an electrocardiogram? If so, when?

Do you have high blood pressure?

Do you have varicose veins, swollen ankles, or intermittent pain in your legs?

Are your legs often cold?

Breasts

Ask women these questions:

Do you perform monthly breast self-examinations?

Have you noticed a lump, a change in breast contour, breast pain, or discharge from your nipples?

– Have you ever had breast cancer? Has anyone in your fami
– Have you ever had a mammogram? If so, when and what
were the results?
- Ask men these questions:
  – Do you have pain in your breast tissue?
  – Have you noticed lumps or a change in
  contour?

GI system

- Have you experienced nausea, vomiting,
loss of appetite, heartburn, abdominal
pain, frequent belching, or passing of gas?
- Have you recently lost or gained weight?
- How often do you have a bowel movement? What is the color, odor,
and consistency of your stools?
- Have you noticed a change in
your usual elimination pattern?
- Do you use laxatives frequently?
- Have you had hemorrhoids, rectal bleeding, hernias, gallbladder
disease, or liver disease?

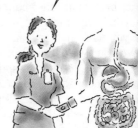

Shed some
light on your
patient's GI
health. Ask abou
elimination
patterns, GI
conditions, and
laxative use.

Genitourinary system

- Do you have urinary problems, such as burning during uri
tion, incontinence, urgency, retention, reduced flow, or dri
bling?
- Do you get up during the night to urinate? If so, how many
times?
- What color is your urine?
- Have you ever noticed blood in your urine?
- Have you ever been treated for kidney stones?

Female reproductive system

- How old were you when you started menstruating?
- How often do you get your period, and how long does it la

Do you have pain or pass clots during your period?

If you're postmenopausal, when did you stop menstruating?

If you're in the transitional stage, what perimenopausal symptoms are you experiencing?

Have you ever been pregnant? If so, how many times? What was the method of each delivery?

How many pregnancies resulted in live births? How many resulted in miscarriages?

Have you had an abortion?

Do you use birth control? If so, what method do you use?

Are you involved in a long-term, monogamous relationship?

Have you had frequent vaginal infections or a sexually transmitted disease?

When was your last gynecologic examination and Pap smear? What were the results?

Male reproductive system

Do you perform monthly testicular self-examinations?

Have you ever had a prostate examination? If so, when?

Have you noticed testicular lumps or penile pain, discharge, or lesions?

Do you use birth control? If so, which form do you use?

Have you had a vasectomy?

Are you involved in a long-term, monogamous relationship?

Have you ever had a sexually transmitted disease?

Musculoskeletal system

Do you have difficulty walking, sitting, or standing?

Are you steady on your feet or do you lose your balance easily?

Do you have arthritis, gout, a back injury, or muscle weakness?

Neurologic system

Have you ever had a seizure?

Are you less able to get around than you think you should be?

Tips for assessing a severely ill patient

When the patient's condition doesn't allow a full assessment—for instance, if the patient is in severe pain—get as much information as possible from other sources. With a severely ill patient, keep these key points in mind:

• Identify yourself to the patient and his family.
• Stay calm to gain the patient's confidence and allay his anxiety.
• Stay on the lookout for important information. For example, if a patient seeks help for a ringing in his ears, don't overlook his casual mention of a periodic "racing heartbeat."
• Avoid jumping to conclusions. Don't assume that the patient's complaint is related to his admitting diagnosis. Use a systematic approach and collect the appropriate information; then draw conclusions.

• Do you ever experience tremors, twitching, numbness, tingling, or loss of sensation in any part of your body?

Endocrine system
• Have you been unusually tired lately?
• Do you feel hungry or thirsty more often than usual?
• Have you lost weight for unexplained reasons?
• How well can you tolerate heat or cold?
• Do you take hormone medications?

Hematologic system
• Have you ever been diagnosed with blood problems?
• Do you bruise easily or become fatigued quickly?
• Have you ever had a blood transfusion? If so, did you have any adverse reactions?

Mental health
• Do you ever experience mood swings or memory loss?
• Do you ever feel anxious, depressed, unable to cope, or unable to concentrate?
• Are you feeling unusually stressed?

Fundamentals of physical assessment

2

Now let's get physical. These are the fundamentals of physical assessment.

INSPECTION
PALPATION
PERCUSSION
AUSCULTATION

Assessment tools

- Stethoscope
  - Diaphragm—flat, thin, plastic surface that picks up high-pitched sounds such as breath sounds
  - Bell—smaller, open end that picks up low-pitched sound such as third and fourth heart sounds
- Penlight to illuminate the inside of the patient's nose and mouth, cast tangential light on lesions, and evaluate pupilla reactions
- Ophthalmoscope to examine the internal structures of the eye
- Otoscope to examine the external auditory canal and tymp ic membrane
- Cotton balls to test sensation
- Safety pins to test pain differentiation
- Percussion hammer to evaluate deep tendon reflexes
- Gloves to protect the patient and you

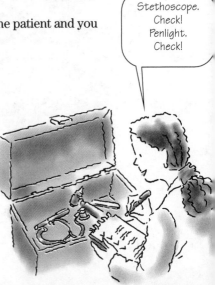

Stethoscope. Check! Penlight. Check!

rforming a general survey

serving the patient

bserve for unusual behavior.

bserve for signs of illness.

paring the patient

troduce yourself to the patient before the assessment, referably when he's dressed.

riefly explain:

what you're planning to do and why

how long it will take

what position changes it will require

what equipment you'll use.

xplain each step in detail as you perform the assessment.

Memory jogger

Use the mnemonic **SOME TEAMS** as a checklist to help you remember what to look for when observing a patient.

mmetry — Are his face and dy symmetrical?

— Does he look his age?

ntal acuity — Is he alert, con-ed, agitated, or inattentive?

ression — Does he appear ill, in n, or anxious?

Trunk — Is he lean, stocky, obese, or barrel-chested?

Extremities — Are his fingers clubbed? Does he have joint abnor-malities or edema?

Appearance — Is he clean and appropriately dressed?

Movement — Are his posture, gait, and coordination normal?

Speech — Is his speech relaxed, clear, strong, understandable, and appropriate? Does he sound stressed?

Recording vital signs and statistics

- Accurate measurements of your patient's height, weight, a[nd] vital signs provide critical information about body functio[n]
- The first time you assess a patient, record his baseline vita[l] signs and statistics.
- Take measurements at regular intervals, depending on the [pa]tient's condition and your facility's policy.
- A series of readings usually provides more valuable inform[a]tion than a single set.

Height and weight

- Height and weight help evaluate nutritional status, calcula[te] medication dosages, and assess fluid loss or gain.
- A baseline can help you gauge future weight changes or ca[l]culate medication dosages in an emergency.

Body temperature

- Body temperature is measured in degrees Fahrenheit (F) [or] degrees Celsius (C).
- Normal body temperature ranges from 96.7° to 100.5° F (3[6]° to 38.1° C), depending on the route used for measurement[.]

Tips for interpreting vital signs

- Analyze all vital signs at the same time, because two or more abnorm[al] values provide important clues to your patient's problem. For example, [a] rapid, thready pulse along with low blood pressure may signal shock.
- If you obtain an abnormal value, take the vital sign again to make sure the reading is accurate.
- Normal readings vary with the patient's age. For example, temperature decreases with age, and respiratory rate may increase with age [or] with an underlying condition.
- An abnormal value for one patient may be a normal value for anoth[er]
- Each patient has his own baseline values, which is why recording vital signs during the initial assessment is so important.

Obtaining pediatric measurements

Height

• Until a child is 2 to 3 years old, measure his height (length) from the top of his head to the bottom of his heel while he's lying down.

• Hold the infant's head in the midline position.

• Hold his knees together with your other hand, gently pressing them down toward the table until fully extended.

• Measure the length. If the infant is active, you may need another person to assist you.

Weight

• If a child is young enough to have his length measured while he's lying down, you'll most likely weigh him on an infant scale.

• Infant scales may be digital or have a balancing arrow.

• While you weigh an infant or a child, he sits or lies in a "bucket" or other enclosed area of the scale.

• To prevent injury to a child, never turn away or leave him unattended on a scale.

• You can usually use an adult scale to weigh older children.

Head circumference

• You'll measure a child's head circumference until he's 3 years old.

• This measurement reflects the growth of the cranium and its contents.

• Place a flexible measuring tape around the child's head at the widest point, from the frontal bone of the forehead and around the occipital prominence at the back of the head.

Hyperthermia is an oral temperature above 106° F (41.1° C). Hypothermia is a rectal temperature below 95° F (35° C).

Pulse

Pulse reflects the amount of blood ejected with each heartbeat. The normal rate for an adult is between 60 and 100 beats/minute. To assess, palpate one of the patient's arterial pulse points and note the rate, rhythm, and amplitude of the pulse. Radial pulse is the most accessible.

How temperature readings compare

Method	Normal temperature	Used with
Oral	97.7° to 99.5° F (36.5° to 37.5° C)	Adults and older children who are awake, alert, and oriented
Axillary (armpit)	96.7° to 98.5° F (35.9° to 36.9° C)	Infants, young children, and patients with impaired immune systems
Rectal	98.7° to 100.5° F (37.1° to 38.1° C)	Infants, young children, and confused or unconscious patients
Tympanic (ear)	98.2° to 100° F (36.8° to 37.8° C)	Adults and children, cooperative patients, and confused or unconscious patients

- Femoral or carotid pulses more accurately reflect the heart activity in a cardiovascular emergency.
- Palpate by using the pads of your index and middle fingers
- Press the area over the artery until you feel pulsations.
- If the rhythm is regular, count the beats for 30 seconds and then multiply by 2 to get the number of beats per minute.
- If the rhythm is irregular, or if your patient has a pacemaker count the beats for 1 minute.
- When taking the patient's pulse for the first time (or when taining baseline data), count the beats for 1 minute.
- Avoid exerting a lot of pressure when palpating the carotid pulse. This can stimulate the vagus nerve and cause reflex bradycardia.

ulse sites

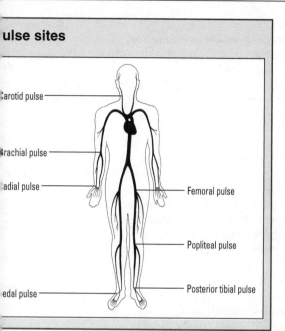

Carotid pulse

Brachial pulse

adial pulse

edal pulse

Femoral pulse

Popliteal pulse

Posterior tibial pulse

on't palpate both carotid pulses at the same time; doing so
an impair cerebral blood flow and function.
the pulse is irregular:
evaluate whether the irregularity follows a pattern
auscultate the apical pulse while palpating the radial pulse
ou should feel the pulse every time you hear a heartbeat).
easure pulse deficit.
Calculate the difference between the apical pulse rate and
e radial pulse rate.
The deficit helps evaluate the ability of each cardiac contrac-
on to eject sufficient blood into the peripheral circulation.
ssess the pulse amplitude by using a numerical scale or de-
riptive term to rate or characterize the strength.
Absent pulse—not palpable, measured as 0

– *Weak* or *thready pulse*—hard to feel, easily obliterated b
slight finger pressure, measured as +1
– *Normal pulse*—easily palpable, obliterated by strong fin
pressure, measured as +2
– *Bounding pulse*—readily palpable, forceful, not easily o
erated by pressure from the fingers, measured as +3

Respirations

- Be aware of the depth and rhythm of each breath.
- Count respirations for 1 minute to determine the rate.
  – Normal respiratory rate for an adult is 16 to 20 breaths/
  minute.
  – Take the patient's respirations while you take his pulse. (
  the patient knows you're counting how often he breathes,
  may subconsciously alter the rate.)
- Watch the patient's chest rise and fall to assess the depth c
  his respirations.
- Observe the rhythm and symmetry of his chest wall as it e
  pands during inspiration and relaxes during expiration.
- Skeletal deformity, fractured ribs, and collapsed lung tissu
  can cause unequal chest expansion.
- Watch for accessory muscle use; patients with chronic obstructive pulmonary disease (COPD) or respiratory distres
  may use neck muscles, including the sternocleidomastoid
  muscles, and abdominal muscles for breathing.
- Check patient position during normal breathing (may indi
  problems such as COPD).
- Normal respirations are quiet and easy; note abnormal
  sounds, such as wheezing and stridor.

Blood pressure

- Systolic reading reflects the maximum pressure exerted o
  the arterial wall at the peak of left ventricular contraction.
  – Normal systolic pressure ranges from 100 to 119 mm Hg.
- Diastolic reading reflects the minimum pressure exerted c
  the arterial wall during left ventricular relaxation.

sing a sphygmomanometer

For accuracy and consistency, sition your patient with his per arm at heart level and his lm turned up.

Apply the cuff snugly, 1″ (2.5 cm) ove the brachial pulse.

Position the manometer at your e level.

Palpate the brachial or radial lse with your fingertips while flating the cuff.

Inflate the cuff to 30 mm Hg ove the point where the pulse sappears.

Place the bell of your stetho-ope over the point where you lt the pulse, as shown in the oto. (Using the bell will help you tter hear Korotkoff's sounds, hich indicate pulse.)

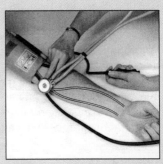

• Release the valve slowly and note the point at which Korotkoff's sounds reappear. The start of the pulse sound indicates the systolic pressure.

• The sounds will become muffled and then disappear. The last Korotkoff's sound you hear is the diastolic pressure.

Normal diastolic pressure ranges from 60 to 79 mm Hg.
A sphygmomanometer is used to measure blood pressure; it onsists of an inflatable cuff, a pressure manometer, and a ulb with a valve.

Blood pressure can be measured from most extremity pulse oints; the brachial artery is used for most patients because f its accessibility.

Performing a physical assessment

- Use drapes so only the area being examined is exposed.
- Develop a pattern for your assessments, starting with the same body system and proceeding in the same sequence.
- Organize your steps to minimize the number of times the patient needs to change position.
- Use inspection, palpation, percussion, and auscultation in sequence except when you perform an abdominal assessment.
- When assessing the abdomen, use the sequence of inspection, auscultation, percussion, and palpation.

Inspection

- Inspect each body system using vision, smell, and hearing to assess normal conditions and deviations.
- Observe color, size, location, movement, texture, symmetry, odors, and sounds as you assess each body system.

Palpation

- Keep your fingernails short, and make sure your hands are warm.
- Always palpate tender areas last.
- Tell your patient the purpose of your touch and what you're feeling with your hands.
- Wear gloves when palpating, especially when palpating mucous membranes or other areas where you might come in contact with body fluids.
- As you palpate each body system, evaluate:
  - texture—rough or smooth?
  - temperature—warm, hot, or cold?
  - moisture—dry, wet, or moist?
  - motion—still or vibrating?
  - consistency of structures—solid or fluid-filled?
  - patient response—pain or tenderness?

Types of palpation

Light palpation
- Use this technique to feel for surface abnormalities.
- Depress the skin ½" to ¾" (1.5 to 2 cm) with your finger pads, using the lightest touch possible.
- Assess for texture, tenderness, temperature, moisture, elasticity, pulsations, superficial organs, and masses.

Deep palpation
- Use this technique to feel internal organs and masses for size, shape, tenderness, symmetry, and mobility.
- Depress the skin 1½" to 2" (4 to 5 cm) with firm, deep pressure.
- Use one hand on top of the other to exert firmer pressure, if needed.

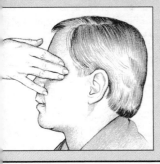
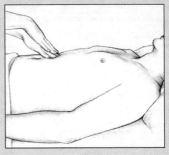

Percussion

- Percussion involves tapping your fingers or hands quickly and sharply against parts of the patient's body, usually the chest or abdomen.
- It helps you locate organ borders and identify organ shape and position.
- It helps determine whether an organ is solid or filled with fluid or gas.
- Depending on their density, organs and tissues produce sounds of varying volume, pitch, and duration.
- *Tympany*, a drumlike sound, is heard over enclosed air and signifies air in the bowel.

Types of percussion

Direct percussion

This technique reveals tenderness; it's commonly used to assess an adult patient's sinuses.
• Using one or two fingers, tap directly on the body part.
• Ask the patient to tell you which areas are painful, and watch his face for signs of discomfort.

Indirect percussion

This technique elicits sounds that give clu to the makeup of the underlying tissue.
• Press the distal part of the middle finger of your nondominant hand firmly on the body part.
• Keep the rest of your hand off the body surface.
• Flex the wrist of your dominant hand.
• Using the middle finger of your dominan hand, tap quickly and directly over the poi where your other middle finger touches th patient's skin.
• Listen to the sounds produced.

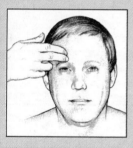
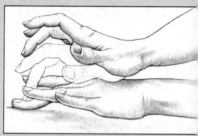

– *Resonance*, a hollow sound, is heard over areas that are p air and part solid, such as the normal lung.
– *Hyperresonance*, a booming sound, is heard over air, as i the lung with emphysema.
– *Dullness*, a thudlike sound, is heard over solid tissue, suc as the liver, spleen, and heart.
– *Flatness*, a flat sound, is heard over dense tissue, such as muscle and bone.
• Compare sounds on one side of the body with those on the other side.

Auscultation

Auscultation involves listening for various breath, heart, and bowel sounds with a stethoscope.

Clean the heads and end pieces of the stethoscope with alcohol or a disinfectant before each use.

Hold the diaphragm of the stethoscope firmly against the patient's skin.

Hold the bell lightly against the patient's skin, just enough to form a seal.

If the patient has hair on his chest, dampen the hair lightly before auscultating to prevent interference from the hair.

Provide a quiet environment.

Expose the area to be auscultated; don't auscultate over a gown or bed linens.

Warm the stethoscope head in your hand before use.

Close your eyes to help focus your attention.

Listen to and try to identify the characteristics of one sound at a time.

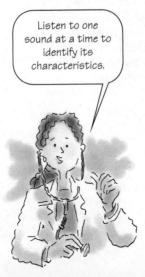

Recording your findings

- Begin your documentation with general information, including the patient's:
  - age
  - race
  - sex
  - general appearance
  - height, weight, and body mass
  - vital signs
  - communication skills
  - behavior
  - awareness and orientation
  - level of cooperation.
- Precisely record all information you obtained using the four physical assessment techniques.
- Follow an organized pattern for recording your findings; document all information about one body system before proceeding to another.
- Use anatomic landmarks in your descriptions so that other people caring for the patient can compare their findings with yours.

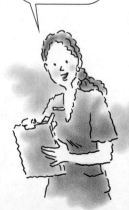

Document your findings in a detailed, yet organized manner.

Nutritional assessment

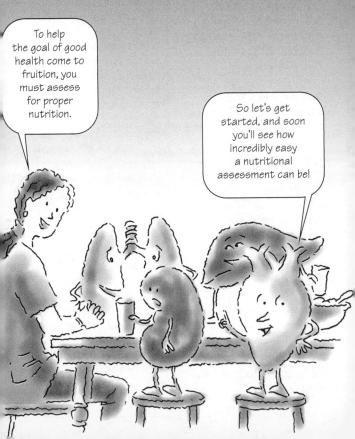

Nutrition overview

- Nutritional health can influence the body's response to illness and treatment.
- Understanding your patient's nutritional status can help you plan his care more effectively.
- Nutrition refers to the sum of the processes by which a living organism:
  - ingests nutrients
  - digests nutrients
  - absorbs nutrients
  - transports nutrients
  - uses nutrients
  - excretes nutrients.
- Types of nutrients include:
  - proteins
  - fats
  - carbohydrates
  - water
  - vitamins
  - minerals.
- For adequate nutrition, a person must:
  - receive the proper nutrients
  - have a properly functioning digestive system for the body to make use of the nutrients.

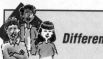

Different strokes

Differences in food intake

What your patient eats depends on cultural and economic influences. Understanding these influences can give you insight into the patient's nutritional status:

- *Socioeconomic status* may affect a patient's ability to buy healthful foods in the quantities needed to maintain proper health. Low socioeconomic status can lead to nutritional problems, especially for small children and pregnant women (who may experience complications during labor or give birth to low-birth-weight infants).
- *Work schedule* can affect the amount and type of food a patient eats, especially if the patient works full-time at night.
- *Religion* can restrict food choices. For example, some Jews and Muslims don't eat pork products, and many Roman Catholics avoid meat on Ash Wednesday and Fridays during Lent.
- *Ethnic background* influences food choices. For example, fish and rice are staple foods for many Asians.

ealth history

Determine the patient's chief complaint, which may include
one or more of these common nutrition-related problems:
weight gain or loss
changes in energy level
changes in appetite or taste
dysphagia
GI tract problems, such as nausea, vomiting, and diarrhea
body system changes, such as skin and nail abnormalities.
Ask the patient about:
previous medical problems
surgical history
current medications (in-
cluding over-the-counter
medications, vitamins,
and herbal preparations)
unusual physical ac-
tivity
weight loss or gain
allergies
smoking
eating patterns
alcohol or drug use
food choices
dietary restrictions
family history of obesity, diabetes, metabolic disorders such
as hypercholesterolemia, and stomach and GI disturbances
(these problems commonly run in families)
his typical day
what and how much he ate yesterday, how the food was
cooked, and who cooked it.

Parts of a nutritional assessment

HEALTH HISTORY

LABORATORY TESTS

BODY SYSTEMS ASSESSMENT

ANTHROPOMETRIC MEASUREMENTS

Physical assessment

- Evaluate the patient's general appearance before starting th physical assessment.
  - Does he look rested?
  - Is his posture good?
  - Is his speech clear?
  - Are his height and weight proportional to his body build?
  - Are his physical movements smooth with no apparent we nesses?
  - Is he free from skeletal deformities?
- Evaluate lab findings as the last step in your assessment .

Body systems

Skin, hair, and nails

- Is the patient's hair shiny and full?
- Is his skin free from blemishes and rashes?
- Is his skin warm and dry, with normal color?
- Are his nails firm with pink beds?

Eyes, nose, throat, and neck

- Are the patient's eyes clear and shiny?
- Are the mucous membranes in his nose moist and pink?
- Is his tongue pink with papillae present?
- Are his gums moist and pink?
- Is his mouth free from ulcers or lesions?
- Is his neck free from masses that would impede swallowin

Cardiovascular system

- Is the patient's heart rhythm regular?
- Are his heart rate and blood pressure normal for his age?
- Are his extremities free from swelling?

Respiratory system

- Are the patient's lungs clear?
- Can he clear his own secretions?
- Is his chest expansion normal during breathing?

system

Is the patient's appetite satisfactory?
Is he free from GI problems?
Are his elimination patterns regular?
Is his abdomen free from abnormal masses on palpation?

Neuromuscular system

Is the patient alert and responsive?
Are his reflexes normal?
Is his behavior appropriate?
Is there evidence of muscle wasting?
Does he have calf pain?
Are his legs and feet free from paresthesia?

Anthropometric measurements

You won't always need to take all measurements, but height and weight are usually necessary.

Measuring height and weight

If your patient can stand without assistance:
- measure his height using the height bar on the scale
- weigh him using a calibrated balance beam scale.
If your patient is weak or bedridden:
- measure his height with a measuring stick or tape
- weigh him using a bed scale.
Ideal body weight refers to standard weights associated with various heights on a reference table.
Weight as a percentage of ideal body weight is obtained by dividing the patient's true weight by an ideal body

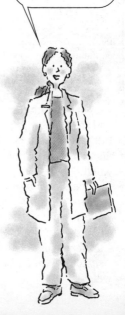

Although not all anthropometric measurements are necessary all the time, it's usually necessary to take height and weight measurements.

Factors affecting nutritional status

Physical condition
- Chronic illnesses (diabetes, for example) and neurologic, cardiac, or thyroid problems
- Family history of diabetes or heart disease
- Draining wounds or fistulas
- Obesity or a weight gain of 20% above normal body weight
- Unplanned weight loss of 20% below normal body weight
- Cystic fibrosis
- History of GI disturbances
- Anorexia or bulimia
- Depression or anxiety
- Severe trauma
- Recent chemotherapy, radiation therapy, or bone marrow transplantation

- Physical limitations, such as paresis or paralysis
- Recent major surgery
- Pregnancy, especially teen or multiple-birth pregnancy
- Burns

Drugs and diet
- Fad diets
- Steroid, diuretic, or antacid use
- Mouth, tooth, or denture problems
- Excessive alcohol intake
- Strict vegetarian diet
- Liquid diet or nothing by mouth for more than 3 days

Lifestyle factors
- Lack of support from family or friends
- Financial problems

---

weight—a number found on an ideal body weight table—and then multiplying that number by 100.
- Body weight that's 120% or more of the ideal body weight indicates obesity; below 90% indicates less-than-adequate weight.
- Key weight categories include:
  – *normal weight*—10% above or below recommended weig
  – *overweight*—10% to 20% above recommended weight
  – *obese*—20% or more above recommended weight
  – *underweight*—10% to 20% below recommended weight
  – *seriously underweight*—20% or more below recommend weight.

Body mass index (BMI) is a measure of body fat based on height and weight.

To determine a patient's BMI, consult a BMI chart or use this formula:

$$BMI = \left(\frac{\text{weight in pounds}}{(\text{height in inches}) \times (\text{height in inches})} \right) \times 703$$

Weight definitions based on BMI are:

underweight—BMI less than 18.5

normal weight—BMI between 18.5 and 24.9

overweight—BMI between 25 and 29.9

obese—BMI of 30 or greater.

Other anthropometric measurements that are used to evaluate muscle mass and subcutaneous fat include:

midarm circumference

midarm muscle circumference

skin-fold thickness.

Laboratory studies

Serum albumin study assesses protein level in the body.

Level is decreased with serious protein deficiency and loss of blood protein resulting from burns, cancer, heart failure, infections, major surgery, malnutrition, or liver or renal disease.

Hemoglobin level helps assess the blood's oxygen-carrying capacity.

Decreased level suggests iron deficiency anemia, protein deficiency, excessive blood loss, or overhydration.

Increased level suggests dehydration or polycythemia.

Hematocrit reflects the proportion of red blood cells in a whole blood sample.

Decreased values suggest iron deficiency anemia, excessive fluid intake, or excessive blood loss.

Increased values suggest severe dehydration or polycythemia.

Taking anthropometric arm measurements

Midarm circumference
Find the arm's midpoint circumference by placing the tape measure halfway between the axilla and the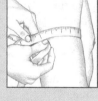
elbow, as shown. Record the measurement in centimeters.

Triceps skin-fold thickness
1. Grasp the patient's skin with your thumb and forefinger, about ⅜″ (1 cm) above the midpoint.
2. Place the calipers at the midpoint and squeeze for 3 seconds, as shown.
3. Record the measurement to the nearest millimeter.

4. Take two more readings and use the average.

Midarm muscle circumference
1. Calculate the midarm muscle circumference by multiplying the triceps skin-fold thickness — measured in millimeters — by 3.14.
2. Subtract this number from the midarm circumference.

Recording the measurements
Record all three measurements a a percentage of the standard me surements, using this formula:

$$\frac{\text{Actual measurement}}{\text{Standard measurement}} \times 100 =$$

A measurement less than 90% the standard indicates caloric deprivation. A measurement greater than 90% indicates adequate or more than adequate energy reserves.

- Serum transferrin level reflects the patient's protein status more accurately than the serum albumin study does.
  - Level decreases along with protein levels, indicating a de tion of protein stores.
  - Decreased values may also indicate inadequate protein pr duction resulting from liver damage, or protein loss from re nal disease, acute or chronic infection, or cancer.

nthropometric measurement values

easurement	Standard	90%
idarm circumference	Men: 29.3 cm Women: 28.5 cm	Men: 26.4 cm Women: 25.7 cm
ceps skin-fold thickness	Men: 12.5 mm Women: 16.5 mm	Men: 11.3 mm Women: 14.9 mm
idarm muscle circumference	Men: 25.3 cm Women: 23.3 cm	Men: 22.8 cm Women: 20.9 cm

Elevated levels may indicate severe iron deficiency.
Jitrogen balance test involves collecting all urine during a 24-
our period.
The test determines the adequacy of a patient's protein in-
ake.
It's the difference between nitrogen intake (determined by a
alorie count done during the same time frame as the 24-hour
rine collection) and excretion.
riglyceride level helps identify hyperlipidemia early.
Increased levels alone aren't diagnostic; further studies,
uch as cholesterol measurements, are required.
Elevated levels occur in patients who consume large
mounts of sugar, soda, and refined carbohydrates.
Decreased levels commonly occur in those who are mal-
ourished.
otal cholesterol test measures circulating levels of free cho-
esterol and cholesterol esters.
Increased levels indicate an increased risk of coronary
rtery disease.
Decreased levels are commonly associated with malnutri-
ion.

Abnormal findings

- Clinical signs of nutritional deficiencies appear late.
- Patients hospitalized for more than 2 weeks are at risk for developing a nutritional disorder.

Excessive weight gain

- Occurs when a person consumes more calories than his body requires for energy
- May result from overeating that's triggered by emotional (such as anxiety, guilt, and depression) and social factors
- Primary sign of many endocrine disorders
- May be caused by activity-limiting conditions, such as cardiovascular or respiratory disorders

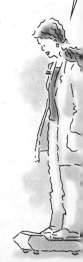

Excessive weight gain may signal a endocrine disorder.

Excessive weight loss

- Usually experienced by patients with nutritional deficiencies
- May result from:
  – decreased food intake, decreased food absorption, increased metabolic requirements, or a combination of the three
  – endocrine, neoplastic, GI, and psychiatric disorders
  – chronic disease
  – infection
  – neurologic lesions that cause paralysis and dysphagia
  – conditions that prevent the patient from consuming a sufficient amount of food, such as painful oral lesions, ill-fitting dentures, or missing teeth

Overweight children

An estimated 15% of children and teens are overweight (based on their body mass index); another 15% risk becoming overweight.

Most overweight children become overweight or obese adults.

Children who are overweight are more likely to have high cholesterol and high blood pressure (risk factors for heart disease) and type 2 diabetes. They also tend to suffer from poor self-esteem and depression because of their weight.

Nursing interventions
• Look for these common causes of excessive weight gain in children:
  – lack of exercise (playing organized sports, riding a bike, or following a regular exercise program)
  – sedentary lifestyle (involving an excessive amount of watching television, using computers, or playing video games)
  – unhealthy eating habits.
• Help the child develop an exercise plan.
• Suggest nutritious eating habits to prevent weight gain and promote a healthy lifestyle.

– poverty
– fad diets
– excessive exercise
– certain drugs

Anorexia

Lack of appetite despite a physiologic need for food
Commonly occurs with GI and endocrine disorders
Can result from anxiety, chronic pain, poor oral hygiene, or changes in taste or smell that normally accompany aging
Can lead to life-threatening malnutrition if chronic
Not to be confused with anorexia nervosa, a psychological condition in which the patient severely restricts food intake, resulting in excessive weight loss

(Text continues on page 42.)

Between the lines

Evaluating nutritional findings

Body system or region	Sign or symptom	Implications
General	• Weakness and fatigue • Weight loss	• Anemia or electrolyte imbalance • Decreased calorie intake, increased calorie use, or inadequate nutrient intake or absorption
Skin, hair, and nails	• Dry, flaky skin • Dry skin with poor turgor • Rough, scaly skin with bumps • Petechiae or ecchymoses • Sore that won't heal • Thinning, dry hair • Spoon-shaped, brittle, or ridged nails	• Vitamin A, vitamin B-complex, or linoleic acid deficiency • Dehydration • Vitamin A or essential fatty acid deficiency • Vitamin C or K deficiency • Protein, vitamin C, or zinc deficiency • Protein or zinc deficiency • Iron deficiency
Eyes	• Night blindness; corneal swelling, softening, or dryness; or Bitot's spots (gray triangular patches on the conjunctiva) • Red conjunctiva	• Vitamin A deficiency • Riboflavin deficiency

Evaluating nutritional findings (continued)

Body system or region	Sign or symptom	Implications
Throat and mouth	• Cracks at corner of mouth	• Riboflavin or niacin deficiency
	• Magenta tongue	• Riboflavin deficiency
	• Beefy, red tongue	• Vitamin B_{12} deficiency
	• Soft, spongy, bleeding gums	• Vitamin C deficiency
	• Swollen neck (goiter)	• Iodine deficiency
Cardiovascular	• Edema	• Protein deficiency
	• Tachycardia and hypotension	• Fluid volume deficit
	• Ascites	• Protein deficiency
Musculoskeletal	• Bone pain and bow leg	• Vitamin D or calcium deficiency
	• Muscle wasting	• Protein, carbohydrate, or fat deficiency
	• Pain in calves and thighs	• Thiamine deficiency
Neurologic	• Altered mental state	• Dehydration and thiamine or vitamin B_{12} deficiency
	• Paresthesia	• Vitamin B_{12}, pyridoxine, or thiamine deficiency

Muscle wasting

- Also known as *atrophy*
- Results from chronic protein deficiency
- Leads to:
  - Loss of muscle fiber bulk and length
  - Shrinkage of and loss of contour in involved muscles, making them appear emaciated or deformed
- Associated with:
  - chronic fatigue
  - apathy
  - anorexia
  - dry skin
  - peripheral edema
  - dull, sparse, dry hair

Mental health assessment

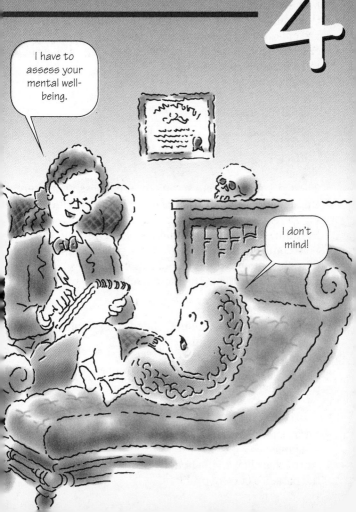

Health history

- Begin your assessment with a health history.
- Establish a therapeutic relationship with the patient that's built on trust.
- Communicate to the patient that his thoughts and behavior are important.
- Effective communication involves speech as well as nonverbal communication, such as:
  - eye contact
  - posture
  - facial expressions
  - gestures
  - clothing
  - affect
  - silence.
- Choose a quiet, private setting for the assessment interview (Interruptions and distractions jeopardize confidentiality and interfere with effective listening.)
- Introduce yourself and explain the interview's purpose.
- Sit a comfortable distance from the patient.
- Give the patient your undivided attention.
- Reorient the patient if he has cognitive or memory loss.
- Be professional but friendly.
- Maintain eye contact.
- Use a calm, nonthreatening tone of voice to encourage the patient to talk more openly.
- Avoid value judgments.
- Don't rush through the interview; building a trusting therapeutic relationship takes time.

Patient interview

- Information obtained during the interview:
  - establishes a baseline
  - provides clues to the underlying or precipitating cause of the patient's current problem.

Therapeutic communication techniques

Listening
Enables you to hear and analyze everything the patient says
Provides insight into the patient's communication patterns

Rephrasing
Involves succinct rephrasing of key patient statements
Helps ensure understanding and recognition of the important points of the patient's message

Broad openings and general statements
Encourage the patient to talk about any subject that comes to mind
Allow the patient to emphasize what seems important to him
Demonstrate a willingness to interact

Clarification
Clarifies a confusing or vague message
Demonstrates a desire to understand what the patient is saying
Elicits precise information crucial to the patient's recovery

Focusing
• Redirects attention to something specific
• Fosters the patient's self-control
• Helps avoid vague generalizations, so the patient can accept responsibility for facing problems

Silence
• Gives the patient time to talk, think, and gain insight into problems
• Provides an opportunity to gather more information
• Must be used judiciously to avoid seeming disinterested or judgmental

Suggesting collaboration
• Gives the patient the opportunity to explore the pros and cons of a suggested approach
• Must be used carefully to avoid directing the patient

Sharing impressions
• Attempts to describe the patient's feelings and then seeks corrective feedback from him
• Allows the patient to clarify misperceptions
• Enables a better understanding of the patient's true feelings

Different strokes

Transcultural communication

- Be aware of cultural differences in communication styles.
- Qualities viewed as desirable in one culture may not be considered appropriate in another culture. For example:
  – Direct eye contact is considered inappropriate and disrespectful i some Asian, Native American, and Arabic-speaking cultures.
  – Some Middle Eastern cultures focus solely on the present; they usually view the future as something to be accepted as it occurs, rather than planned.
  – Some Asians strongly value harmonious interpersonal relationships. To maintain harmony, they may nod, smile, and provide answers they feel are expected rather than expressing their true feelings and concerns.

- A patient with a mental illness or other mental impairment may not be a reliable source of information.
  – Check hospital records for previous admissions.
  – Compare the patient's past and present behavior, sympto and circumstances.

Chief complaint

- The patient may not directly voice his chief complaint; you others may note that he's having difficulty coping or that h exhibiting unusual behavior.
- If you note a problem, determine whether the patient is aw of it.
- Document the patient's response word for word and enclos it in quotation marks.
- Inquire about symptoms, including:
  – severity and persistence
  – whether they occurred suddenly or developed over time.

story of psychiatric illnesses

Discuss past psychiatric disturbances, including:
- delusions
- violence
- suicide attempts
- drug or alcohol abuse
- depression.

Discuss previous psychiatric treatment, if any.

Ask about any family history of psychiatric illness or substance abuse.

mographic data

Obtain demographic data to establish a baseline and confirm that the patient's record is correct, including:
- age
- ethnic origin
- primary language
- birthplace
- religion
- occupation
- marital status.

cioeconomic data

Patients suffering hardships are more likely to show symptoms of distress during an illness.

Educational level, family, housing conditions, income, and employment status may provide clues to the patient's current problem.

ltural and religious beliefs

Background and values can affect how the patient responds to illness and adapts to care.

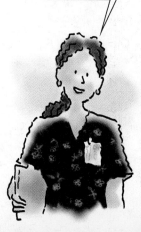

Socioeconomic factors such as educational level, income, and employment status may provide clues to the patient's current problem.

- Certain questions and behaviors considered acceptable in ⟨ culture may be inappropriate in another.

Medication history

- Medications can cause symptoms of mental illness.
- Review medications the patient is taking, including over-th counter and herbal preparations, and check for interaction
- If the patient is taking a psychiatric drug, ask these questio
  - Have your symptoms improved?
  - Are you taking the medication as prescribed?
  - Have you had any adverse reactions?

Physical illnesses

- Determine whether the patient has a history of medical dis ders that may cause distorted thought processes, disorient tion, depression, or other symptoms of mental illness, such as:
  - renal or hepatic failure
  - infection
  - thyroid disease
  - stroke
  - metabolic disorder.

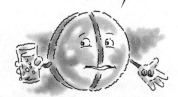

I don't do it on purpose, but in addition to treating a particular condition, I may cause symptoms of mental illness.

ntal status assessment

ost of a mental status assessment can be done during an in-
rview.

ssess:
 appearance
 behavior
 mood
 thought processes
 cognitive function
 coping mechanisms
 potential for self-destructive behavior.
ecord your findings.

ial observations

pearance

ote the patient's dress and grooming.
 Is he clean?
 Is his appearance appropriate for his age, sex, and situation.
 heck whether his posture is erect or slouched.
 ote whether his head is lowered.
 bserve his gait.
 Is it brisk, slow, shuffling, or unsteady?
 ote his facial expression.
 Does he look alert or stare blankly?
 Does he appear sad or angry?
 Does he maintain eye contact?
 Does he stare at you for long periods?

avior

ote the patient's demeanor and overall attitude.
 ote extraordinary behavior such as speaking to a person
ho isn't present.
 ecord his mannerisms.
 Does he bite his nails, fidget, or pace?
 Does he display tics or tremors?

– How does he respond to you?
– Is he cooperative, friendly, hostile, or indifferent?

Mood

- Note whether the patient appears anxious or depressed.
  – Is he crying, sweating, breathing heavily, or trembling?
- Ask him to describe his current feelings in concrete terms and to suggest possible reasons for these feelings.
- Note inconsistencies between body language and mood (s as smiling when discussing an anger-provoking situation).

Thought processes and cognitive function

- Evaluate the patient's orientation to time, place, and perso Note any confusion or disorientation.
- Listen for an indication that the patient might be having delusions, hallucinations, obsessions, compulsions, fantasies, or daydreams.
- Assess the patient's attention span and ability to recall events in both the distant and recent past.
- Test intellectual functioning by asking the patient to add a series of numbers.
- Test sensory perception and coordination by having the patient copy a simple drawing.
- Inappropriate responses to questions about a hypothetical situation (for example, "What would you do if you won the lottery?") can indicate impaired judgment. Keep in mind that the patient's cultural background will influence his answers.
- Note speech characteristics that may indicate altered thought processes, including:
  – monosyllabic responses

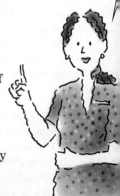

Pay attention to th patient's speec characteristic because they m indicate altere thought processes.

- irrelevant or illogical replies to questions
- convoluted or excessively detailed speech
- slurred speech
- repetitious speech patterns
- flight of ideas
- sudden silence without obvious reason.

Assess insight.
- Does the patient understand the significance of his illness, the treatment plan, and the effect the illness will have on his life?

Coping mechanisms

The patient who's faced with a stressful situation may adopt coping, or defense, mechanisms — behaviors that operate on an unconscious level to protect the ego.

Listen for an excessive reliance on coping mechanisms.

Common coping mechanisms

Denial — the refusal to admit truth or reality

Displacement — transferring an emotion from its original object to a substitute

Fantasy — the creation of unrealistic or improbable images to escape from daily pressures and responsibilities

Identification — the unconscious adoption of another person's personality characteristics, attitudes, values, and behaviors

Projection — the displacement of negative feelings onto another person

Rationalization — the substitution of acceptable reasons for the real or actual reasons motivating behavior

Reaction formation — behaving in a manner opposite from the way the person feels

Regression — the return to behavior of an earlier, more comfortable time

Repression — the exclusion of unacceptable thoughts and feelings from the conscious mind, leaving them to operate in the subconscious

Potential for self-destructive behavior

- Patients who are self-destructive take life-threatening risks
- Not all self-destructive behavior is suicidal in intent.
  – Some patients engage in self-destructive behavior becaus(e) makes them feel alive.
  – The patient may cut or mutilate body parts to focus on physical pain, which may be less overwhelming than emoti(on) al distress.
- Assess for suicidal tendencies, particularly if the patient re(-) ports symptoms of depression.
  – The incidence of suicide is higher in depressed patients th(an) in patients with other diagnoses.
  – If the patient is actively planning suicide, be prepared to ta(ke) immediate action to prevent him from carrying out his plan(.)

Psychological and mental status testing

- Most of a mental status assessment can be done during an (in)terview.
- Other aspects of mental health can be assessed using psyc(ho)logical and mental status tests.
  – *Mini-Mental Status Examination* measures orientation, registration, recall, calculation, language, and graphomoto(r) function.
  – *Cognitive Capacity Screening Examination* measures o(ri)entation, memory, calculation, and language.
  – *Cognitive Assessment Scale* measures orientation, gener(al) knowledge, mental ability, and psychomotor function.
  – *Beck Depression Inventory* helps diagnose depression, d(e)termine its severity, and monitor the patient's response dur(ing) treatment.
  – *Global Deterioration Scale* assesses and stages primary (de)generative dementia based on orientation, memory, and ne(u)rologic function.
  – *Minnesota Multiphasic Personality Inventory* helps ass(ess) personality traits and ego function in adolescents and adul(ts).

bnormal findings

normal thought processes

Derailment — Speech vacillates from one subject to another unrelated one.

Flight of ideas — The patient jumps abruptly from topic to topic in a continuous flow of speech.

Neologisms — Words are distorted or invented.

Confabulation — The patient fabricates facts or events to fill in the gaps where memory loss has occurred.

Clanging — The patient chooses a word based on the sound rather than the meaning.

Echolalia — The patient repeats words or phrases that others say.

Incoherence — The patient's speech is incomprehensible.

> **Memory jogger**
>
> To remember the difference between derailment and flight of ideas, think of the following analogies:
>
> *Derailment* — thoughts get "off track," like a derailed train.
>
> *Flight of ideas* — ideas fly quickly from one topic to another, like a plane flies quickly from one location to another.

normal thought content

Obsessions — recurrent, uncontrollable thoughts, images, or impulses that the patient considers unacceptable

Compulsions — repetitive behaviors that result from attempts to alleviate an obsession

Phobia — an irrational fear of objects or situations

Depersonalization — feeling of detachment from the mind or body or the loss of identity

Delusions — false, fixed beliefs that aren't shared by others

Poverty of content — thoughts that give little information because of vagueness, empty repetition, or obscure phrases

Between the lines

Evaluating mental health findings

Disorder	Assessment findings
Schizophrenia	• Delusions • Hallucinations • Disorganized speech • Grossly disorganized or catatonic behavior • Flat affect • Inability to speak • Poor eye contact • Distant and unresponsive facial expression • Limited body language
Major depressive disorder	• Severe fatigue • Inability to concentrate or make decisions • Feelings of sadness, worthlessness, or extreme gu[...] • Appetite changes with either weight loss or gain • Sleep disturbances • Decreased libido
Bipolar I disorder	• Signs and symptoms of major depressive disorder (listed above) • Manic findings, such as delusions of grandeur, flig[...] of ideas, extreme talkativeness, being easily distract[...] spending money recklessly, or experiencing euphori[...] or irritability

Perception abnormalities

• Perception abnormalities include:
  – *illusions*—misinterpretations of external stimuli
  – *hallucinations*—auditory, visual, tactile, somatic, or gus[...] tory sensory perceptions when no external stimuli are pres[...]

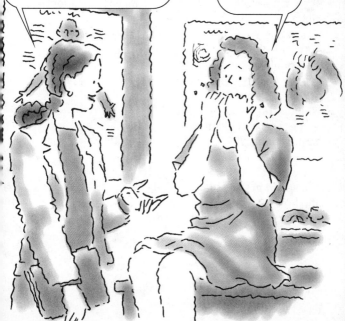

Health history

- Explore the patient's chief complaint, medical history, family history, psychological history, and patterns of daily living.
- Skin, hair, and nail abnormalities may result from a medical problem related to the patient's chief complaint, but the patient may overlook or minimize them.

Asking about the skin

- Most complaints about the skin involve:
  - itching
  - rashes
  - lesions
  - pigmentation abnormalities
  - changes in existing lesions.
- Typical questions to ask about changes in a patient's skin include:
  - How and when did the skin changes occur?
  - Are the changes in the form of a skin rash or lesion?
  - Is the change confined to one area, or has the condition spread?
  - Does the area bleed or have drainage?
  - Does the area itch?
  - How much time do you spend in the sun, and how do you protect your skin from ultraviolet rays?
  - Do you have allergies?
  - Do you have a family history of skin cancer or other significant diseases?

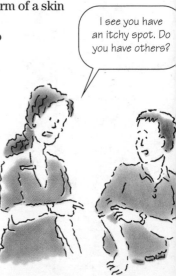

I see you have an itchy spot. Do you have others?

- Do you have a fever or joint pain, or have you lost weight?
- Have you had a recent insect bite?
- Do you take any medications or herbal preparations? If so, which ones?
- What changes in your skin have you observed in the past few years?

Asking about the hair

Concerns about the hair commonly involve hair loss or *hirsutism,* which is an increased growth and distribution of body hair.

Hair loss or hirsutism can be caused by such factors as:
- skin infections
- ovarian or adrenal tumors
- increased stress
- systemic diseases, such as hypothyroidism and malignancies.

Identify the cause of your patient's hair problem by asking:
- When did you first notice the loss (or gain) of hair? Was it sudden or gradual?
- Did the change occur in just a few spots or all over your body?
- What was happening in your life when the problem started?

Additional questions for parents

Does the child have any birthmarks?

When the child was a neonate, did he experience any change in skin color — for example, cyanosis or jaundice?

Have you noted any rashes, burns, or bruises? If so, where and when, and what was the cause?

Has the child been exposed to any contagious skin conditions — such as scabies, lice, or impetigo—or to any other communicable diseases?

– Are you taking any medications or herbal preparations? If so, which ones?
– Are you experiencing itching, pain, discharge, fever, or weight loss?
– What serious illnesses, if any, have you had?

Asking about the nails

- Complaints about the nails commonly concern changes in growth or color that may result from:
  – infection
  – nutritional deficiencies
  – systemic illnesses
  – stress.
- Questions to ask about changes in a patient's nails include:
  – When did you first notice the changes in your nails?
  – What types of changes have you noticed (for example, nail shape, color, or brittleness)?
  – Were the changes sudden or gradual?
  – Do you have other signs or symptoms, such as bleeding, pain, itching, or discharge?
  – What's the normal condition of your nails?
  – Do you have a history of serious illness?
  – Do you have a history of nail problems?
  – Do you bite your nails?
  – Have you had nail tips attached?

Physical assessment

Use inspection and palpation.
Make sure the room is well lit and comfortably warm before beginning your examination.
Wear gloves during your examination.

Skin

Gather the following equipment before beginning your skin assessment:
- clear ruler with centimeter and millimeter markings
- tongue blade
- penlight or flashlight
- Wood's lamp
- magnifying glass.

Observe the skin's overall appearance.
Inspect and palpate the skin area by area.

Color

Look for localized areas of bruising, cyanosis, pallor, and erythema.
Check for uniformity of color and hypopigmented or hyperpigmented areas.
Areas that are exposed to the sun may show a darker pigmentation than other areas.
Color changes may vary depending on skin pigmentation.
In certain cultures, local changes are normal variations.

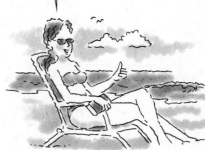

Exposure to the sun usually means darker skin pigmentation.

Different strokes

Detecting color variations in dark-skinned people

Cyanosis
Examine the conjunctivae, palms, soles, buccal mucosa, and tongue. Look for dull, dark color.

Edema
Examine the area for decreased color, and palpate for tightness.

Erythema
Palpate the area for warmth.

Jaundice
Examine the sclerae and hard palate in natural (not fluorescent) light, i⁺ possible. Look for a yellow color.

Pallor
Examine the sclerae, conjunctivae, buccal mucosa, tongue, lips, nail beds, palms, and soles. Look for an ashen color.

Petechiae
Examine areas of lighter pigmentation such as the abdomen. Look for tiny, purplish red dots.

Rashes
Palpate the area for skin texture changes.

Texture and turgor
- Inspect and palpate skin texture, noting its thickness and m⁻ bility; it should look smooth and be intact.
- Rough, dry skin is common with hypothyroidism, psoriasis, and excessive keratinization.
- Skin that isn't intact may indicate local irritation or trauma.
- Palpation helps evaluate hydration status.

Different strokes

Mongolian spots

- Irregularly shaped areas of deep-blue pigmentation
- Most commonly appear over the sacral and gluteal areas; may also appear on the shoulders, arms, abdomen, or thighs
- Are normal variations of the skin in children of African, Asian, or Latin American descent
- Occur in 90% of Black children and 80% of Asian children
- Are present at birth and usually remain visible into adulthood but may fade over time
- Result from deposits of embryonic pigment in the epidermal layer left behind from fetal development
- Are completely benign and require no treatment
- May be confused with bruises, which can cause an erroneous suspicion of child abuse

- Dehydration and edema cause poor skin turgor; however, because aging may also cause poor skin turgor, it isn't a reliable indicator of hydration status in elderly patients.
- Overhydration causes skin to appear edematous and spongy.
- Localized edema can result from trauma or systemic disease.

Moisture

- Skin should be relatively dry, with minimal perspiration.
- Skin-fold areas should be fairly dry.
- Overly dry skin appears red and flaky.
- Overly moist skin can be caused by anxiety, obesity, or an environment that's too warm.
- Heavy sweating, or diaphoresis, usually accompanies:
  - fever
  - strenuous activity
  - cardiac, pulmonary, and other diseases
  - any activity or illness that elevates metabolic rate.

Evaluating skin turgor

• When assessing an adult, gently squeeze the skin on the forearm or sternal area between your thumb and forefinger, as shown at right.
• When assessing an infant, roll a fold of loosely adherent abdominal skin between your thumb and forefinger and then release it.
• If the skin quickly returns to its original shape, the patient has normal turgor.
• If the skin returns to its original shape slowly over 30 seconds or maintains a tented position, as shown at right, the skin has poor turgor.

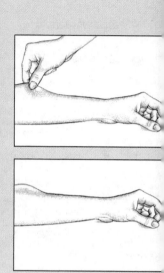

Temperature
• Palpate the skin bilaterally.
• Warm skin suggests normal circulation.
• Cool skin suggests a possible underlying disorder.
• Localized skin coolness can result from vasoconstriction associated with cold environments or impaired arterial circulation to a limb.
• General coolness can result from shock or hypothyroidism.
• Localized warmth occurs in areas that are infected, inflamed or burned.
• Generalized warmth occurs with fever or systemic diseases such as hyperthyroidism.

Lesions
• Normal skin variations include:

birthmarks — generally flat and ange in color from tan to red or rown; found on all areas of the ody

freckles — small, flat macules, sually red-brown or brown; locatd primarily on the face, arms, and ack

nevi — either flat or raised and aay be pink, tan, or dark brown; ound on all areas of the body

moles — flat or slightly elevated nd evenly pigmented; usually tan o dark brown; found on all areas f the body.

ed lesions caused by vascular hanges that may indicate disease iclude:

hemangiomas

telangiectases

petechiae

purpura

ecchymoses.

rimary lesion is a new lesion. econdary lesion results from hanges in a primary lesion. xamples include:

fissures

scales

crusts

scars

excoriations.

se a flashlight or penlight to etermine whether a lesion is olid or fluid-filled.

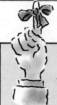

Memory jogger

When assessing subtle skin temperature differences, remember the phrase "subtle D." Use the "d"orsal surfaces of your hands and fingers to detect "subtle" temperature differences between one area of the body and another. They're the most sensitive to changes in temperature.

A penlight can help you determine whether a lesion is solid or fluid-filled.

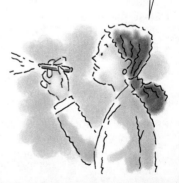

Identifying primary lesions

Macule
Flat, circumscribed area of altered skin color, generally less than 1 cm in diameter; examples: freckle and flat nevus

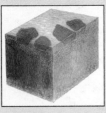

Papule
Raised, circumscribed, solid area; generally less than 1 cm in diameter; examples: elevated nevus or wart

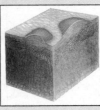

Vesicle
Circumscribed, elevated lesion; contain serous fluid; less tha 1 cm in diameter; example: early chick enpox

– Macules, papules, nodules, wheals, and hives are solid lesions.

– Vesicles, bullae, pustules, and cysts are fluid-filled lesions
- Use a Wood's lamp to identify lesions that fluoresce.
  – Darken the room and shine the light on the lesion.
  – If the lesion looks bluish green, the patient has a fungal ir fection.
- Describe the lesion's characteristics, pattern, location, and distribution.
- Examine the lesion to see whether it looks the same on bo sides.
- Check the borders to see whether they're regular or irregu
  – An asymmetrical lesion with an irregular border may indi cate malignancy.
- Watch for color changes that occur over time.
  – A mole may change from tan or brown to multiple shades tan, dark brown, and black, or a mixture of red, white, and blue.

Help desk

Illuminating lesions

Illuminating a lesion can help you see it better and learn more about its characteristics. Here are two techniques worth perfecting. Before you begin, reduce the direct lighting.

Macule or papule?
Shine a penlight or flashlight at a right angle to the lesion.
If the light casts a shadow, the lesion is a papule.
Macules are flat and don't produce shadows.

Solid or fluid-filled?
Place the tip of a flashlight or penlight against the side of the lesion.
Solid lesions don't transmit light.
Fluid-filled lesions transilluminate with a red glow.

- Color changes may indicate malignancy.
- Look at the configuration and distribution of the lesions; many skin diseases have typical configuration patterns.
- Measure the diameter of the lesion using a millimeter-centimeter ruler.
- An increase in the size or elevation of a mole over many years is common and probably normal.
- Note moles that rapidly change size, especially moles that are ⅛" (6 mm) or larger.
- When documenting lesions, include the type, color and, if any, the odor and amount of drainage.

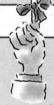

Memory jogger

To remember what to assess when evaluating a lesion, think of the first five letters of the alphabet:

Asymmetry

Border

Color and **C**onfiguration

Diameter and **D**rainage

Evolution or progression of the lesion.

Common lesion configurations

Discrete
Individual lesions are separate and distinct.

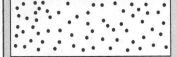

Annular
Lesions are arranged in a single ring or circle.

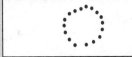

Grouped
Lesions are clustered together.

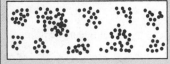

Polycyclic
Lesions are arranged in multiple circles.

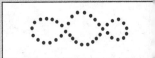

Confluent
Lesions merge so that individual lesions aren't visible or palpable.

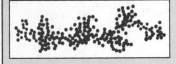

Arciform
Lesions form arcs or curves.

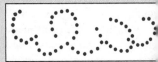

Linear
Lesions form a line.

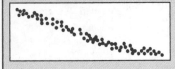

Reticular
Lesions form a meshlike network

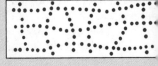

Hair

- Inspect and palpate the hair over the patient's entire body.
- Note the distribution, quantity, texture, and color.

- Hair should be evenly distributed over the entire body.
- Check for patterns of hair loss and growth.
- If the patient has patchy hair loss, look for regrowth.
- Examine the scalp for erythema, scaling, and encrustation.
- Excessive hair loss with scalp crusting may indicate ringworm infestation.
- Check for scalp crusting using a Wood's lamp.
- Note areas of excessive hair growth, which may indicate a hormone imbalance or may be a sign of a systemic disorder such as Cushing's syndrome.
- Hair should be shiny and smooth, not dry or brittle.

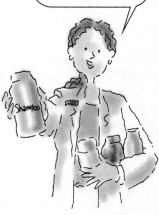

Reviving dry or brittle hair may be as simple as avoiding certain hair care products.

- Dryness or brittleness can result from the use of harsh hair treatments or hair care products or can be caused by a systemic illness.
- Extreme oiliness is usually related to excessive sebum production or poor grooming habits.

Nails

- Examine the color of the nails.
- Light-skinned people generally have pinkish nails.
- Dark-skinned people generally have brown nails.
- Brown-pigmented bands in the nail beds are normal in dark-skinned people and abnormal in light-skinned people.
- Nicotine stains may cause yellow nails in smokers.
- Check nail beds to assess a patient's peripheral circulation.
- Press on the nail bed and then release, noting how long the color takes to return.

– Color should return immediately or within 3 seconds.
- Inspect the shape and contour of the nails.
  – Surface of the nail bed should be either slightly curved or flat.
  – Edges of the nail should be smooth, rounded, and clean.
- Check the angle of the nail base; it's normally less than 180 degrees.
  – An increase in the nail angle suggests clubbing.
  – Curved nails are a normal variation; they may appear to be clubbed until you notice that the nail angle is less than 180 degrees.
- Palpate the nail bed to check the thickness of the nail and the strength of its attachment to the bed.

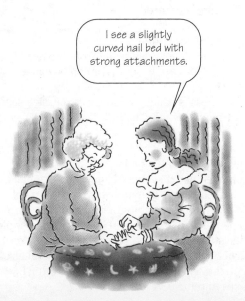

Abnormal findings

Document all abnormal findings, pertinent health history, and as much information as possible from the physical examination.

Skin abnormalities

Café-au-lait spots

Flat, light brown, uniformly hyperpigmented macules or patches on the skin surface

Usually appear during the first 3 years of life but may develop at any age

Differentiated from freckles and other benign birthmarks by their larger size and irregular shape

Usually have no significance

If six or more, may be associated with an underlying neurologic disorder such as neurofibromatosis

Cherry angiomas

Tiny, bright-red, round papules that may become brown over time

Are clinically insignificant

Occur in virtually everyone older than age 30 and increase in number with age

Papular rash

Small, raised, circumscribed (perhaps with shades of red to purple discoloration) lesions known as *papules*

May erupt anywhere on the body in various configurations

May be acute or chronic

Characterize skin disorders

May result from allergy and from infectious, neoplastic, and systemic disorders

Port-wine hemangiomas

Commonly called *port-wine stains*

(Text continues on page 73.)

Between the lines

Evaluating skin, hair, and nail findings

Sign or symptom and findings	Probable cause

Alopecia

• Patchy alopecia, typically on the lower extremities • Thin, shiny, atrophic skin • Thickened nails • Weak or absent peripheral pulses • Cool extremities • Paresthesia	Arterial insufficiency
• Translucent, charred, or ulcerated skin • Pain	Burns
• Loss of the outer third of the eyebrows • Thin, dull, coarse, brittle hair on the face • Fatigue • Constipation • Cold intolerance • Weight gain • Puffy face, hands, and feet	Hypothyroidism

Clubbing

• Anorexia • Malaise • Dyspnea • Tachypnea • Diminished breath sounds • Pursed-lip breathing • Barrel chest • Peripheral cyanosis	Emphysema

valuating skin, hair, and nail findings *(continued)*

gn or symptom and findings	Probable cause
lubbing *(continued)*	
Wheezing Dyspnea Fatigue Neck vein distention Palpitations Unexplained weight gain Dependent edema Crackles on auscultation	Heart failure
Hemoptysis Dyspnea Wheezing Chest pain Fatigue Weight loss Fever	Lung and pleural cancer
ruritus	
Intense, severe pruritus Erythematous rash on dry skin at flexion oints Possible edema, scaling, and pustules	Atopic dermatitis
Scalp excoriation from scratching Matted, foul-smelling, lusterless hair Occipital and cervical lymphadenopathy Oval, gray-white nits on hair shafts	Pediculosis capitis (head lice)

(continued)

Evaluating skin, hair, and nail findings *(continued)*

Sign or symptom and findings	Probable cause
Pruritus *(continued)* • Gradual or sudden pruritus • Ammonia breath odor • Oliguria or anuria • Fatigue • Irritability • Muscle cramps	Chronic renal failure
Urticaria • Rapid eruption of diffuse urticaria and angioedema, with wheals ranging from pinpoint to palm-sized or larger • Pruritic, stinging lesions • Profound anxiety • Weakness • Shortness of breath • Nasal congestion • Dysphagia • Warm, moist skin	Anaphylaxis
• Nonpitting, nonpruritic edema of an extremity of the face • Possibly acute laryngeal edema	Hereditary angioedema
• Erythema chronicum migrans that results in urticaria • Constant malaise and fatigue • Fever • Chills • Lymphadenopathy • Neurologic and cardiac abnormalities • Arthritis	Lyme disease

Usually present at birth
Commonly appear on the face and upper body as flat purple marks

Pruritus

Unpleasant itching sensation
Most common symptom of skin disorders
May result from:
- local or systemic disorder
- drug use
- emotional upset
- contact with skin irritants
May be exacerbated by:
- increased skin temperature
- poor skin turgor
- local vasodilation
- dermatoses
- stress

Purpuric lesions

Caused by red blood cells and blood pigments in the skin
Don't blanch under pressure
Can be classified into three types
- Petechiae — red or brown pinpoint lesions generally caused by capillary fragility; can be caused by diseases associated with the formation of microemboli or bleeding, such as subacute bacterial endocarditis and thrombocytopenia
- Ecchymoses — blue- or purple-tinged discolorations resulting from blood accumulation in the skin after injury to the vessel walls
- Hematomas — masses of blood that accumulate in a tissue, organ, or body space after a break in a blood vessel

Telangiectases

Permanently dilated, small blood vessels that typically form a weblike pattern
Include spider hemangiomas

– Small, red lesions arranged in a weblike configuration
– Usually appear on the face, neck, and chest
– May be normal or associated with pregnancy or cirrhosis

Urticaria

- Also called *hives*
- Vascular skin reaction
- Characterized by the eruption of transient pruritic wheals– smooth, slightly elevated patches with well-defined erythentous margins and pale centers of various shapes and sizes
- Produced by the local release of histamine or other vasoactive substances as part of a hypersensitivity reaction, commonly to:
  – certain drugs
  – foods
  – insect bites
  – inhalants
  – contact with certain substances
- May also result from emotional stress or environmental factors

Vesicular rash

- Scattered or linear distribution of blisterlike lesions
  – Sharply circumscribed
  – Filled with clear, cloudy, or bloody fluid
  – Usually measure less than ⅛″ (6 mm) in diameter
  – May occur singly or in groups
  – Sometimes occur with bullae, fluid-filled lesions larger than ⅛″ in diameter
- May be mild or severe and temporary or permanent
- Can result from infection, inflammation, or allergic reactions

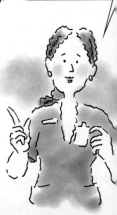

Urticaria typically occurs as part of a hypersensitivity reaction.

Hair abnormalities

Alopecia

- Found more commonly and extensively in men than in women
- Involves diffuse hair loss (usually a normal part of aging)
- May occur as a result of:
  - pyrogenic infections
  - chemical trauma
  - ingestion of certain drugs
  - endocrinopathy and other disorders
- May appear as patchy hair loss caused by:
  - tinea capitis
  - trauma
  - third-degree burns

Hirsutism

- Excessive hairiness in women
- Can develop on the body and face
- May occur locally in pigmented nevi
- Can result from:
  - certain drug therapies
  - endocrine problems, such as Cushing's syndrome and acromegaly

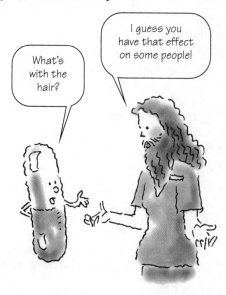

Nail abnormalities

Beau's lines

- Transverse depressions in the nail that extend to the nail bed

- Occur with:
  - acute illness
  - malnutrition
  - anemia
  - trauma that temporarily impairs nail function
- Appear first at the cuticle and then move forward as the na
  grows

Clubbing

- Results when proximal edge of the nail elevates so the angl
  is greater than 180 degrees
- Appears as a thickened nail that's curved at the end with a
  rounder and wider-than-normal distal phalanx

Koilonychia

- Thin, spoon-shaped nails that are white and opaque with la
  eral edges that tilt upward, forming a concave profile
- Associated with:
  - hypochromic anemia
  - chronic infections
  - Raynaud's disease
  - malnutrition

Onycholysis

- Loosening of the nail plate with separation from the nail be
  beginning at the distal groove
- Associated with:
  - minor trauma to long fingernails
  - such disease processes as psoriasis, contact dermatitis, h
    perthyroidism, and *Pseudomonas* infections

Terry's nails

- Transverse bands of white that cover the nail, except for a
  narrow zone at the distal end
- Associated with hypoalbuminemia

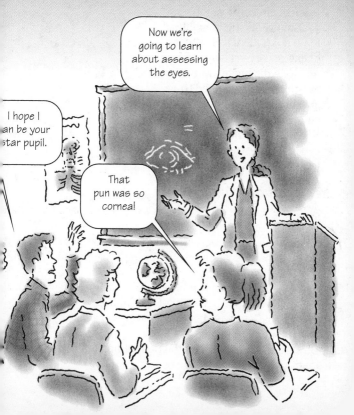

Health history

- Obtain a health history of the eyes.
- The most common eye-related complaints are:
  – diplopia (double vision)
  – visual floaters
  – photobia (light sensitivity)
  – vision loss
  – eye pain.
- Other complaints include:
  – decreased visual acuity or clarity
  – defects in color vision
  – difficulty seeing at night.
- Even if a patient's chief complaint isn't eye-related and previous diagnoses weren't eye-related, you'll need to question him about his eyes and vision.
- Keep in mind that poor vision can affect the patient's ability to comply with treatment.

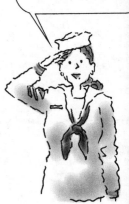

Aye-aye captain! I'll ask the patient about his eyes and vision, even if his chief complaint isn't eye-related.

Asking about the eyes

- Ask whether the patient wears corrective lenses for distant vision or for reading.
- Ask whether he experiences blurred vision, blind spots, floaters, double vision, pain, discharge, or unusual sensitivity to light.
- Ask whether he has trouble seeing at night.
- Obtain the patient's history of eye injuries or eye surgery.
- Ask the patient whether he has ever had a lazy eye.
- Ask about allergies.
- Be sure to find out when the patient had his last eye examination.

sking about general health

Ask the patient about a history of hypertension, diabetes, stroke, multiple sclerosis, syphilis, or human immunodeficiency virus (HIV).

Ask whether family members have glaucoma, cataracts, vision loss, or retinitis; family history may predispose the patient to these conditions, so he'll need frequent testing.

Ask the patient which medications he takes.

- Be aware that some drugs can affect vision; for example, digoxin overdose can cause a patient to see yellow halos round bright lights.

- Ask about over-the-counter drugs, herbal preparations, eyedrops, and eyewashes.

Ask the patient what kind of work he does and what he does or recreation.

- Is he exposed to chemicals, fumes, flying debris, or infectious agents?

- If he's exposed to agents, does he wear eye protection?

Warn patients who smoke that smoking increases the risk of vascular disease, which can lead to blindness.

If your patient is visually impaired or elderly:

- Ask him how well he can manage activities of daily living.

- Assess whether the patient and his family need assistance in learning to use adaptive devices.

- Assess whether he needs a referral to an agency that helps visually impaired people.

When obtaining a young child's health history:

- you'll likely ask the parents the questions

- you may receive only objective answers, not subjective responses.

Help desk

Questions for children and aging adults

Young ones

If your patient is a child, ask his parents these questions:

• Was he delivered vaginally or by cesarean delivery? If he was delivered vaginally, did his mother have a vaginal infection at the time? (Inform the parents that infections such as chlamydia, gonorrhea, genital herpes, or candidiasis can cause eye problems in infants.)

• Did he have erythromycin ointment instilled in his eyes at birth?

• Has he had an eye examination before? If so, when was the most recent examination?

• Has he passed age-appropriate developmental milestones?

• Does he know how to hold and care for sharp objects such as scissors?

Oldies but goodies

If your patient is an aging adult, ask him these questions:

• Have you had any difficulty climbing stairs or driving?

• Have you ever been tested for glaucoma? If so, when and what was the result?

• If you have glaucoma, has your doctor prescribed eyedrops for you? If so, what kind?

• How well can you put drops in your eyes?

• Do your eyes ever feel dry? Do they burn? If so, how do you treat the problem?

ysical assessment

. complete eye assessment involves:
inspecting the external eye and the eyelid
testing visual acuity
assessing eye muscle function
palpating the nasolacrimal sac
examining intraocular structures with an ophthalmoscope.
efore starting your examination, gather the necessary equip-
ent, including:
a good light source
penlight
one or two opaque cards
ophthalmoscope
vision-test cards
gloves
tissues
cotton balls.
[ake sure that the patient is seated comfortably at eye level
ith you.

pecting the eyes

bserve the patient's face.
sing the scalp line as the starting point, check that his eyes
·e in a normal position; they should be about one-third of the
·ay down the face with about one eye-width between them.

·lid

·ach upper eyelid should cover the top quarter of the iris, and
·e eyes should look alike.
Check for an excessive amount of visible sclera above the
·nbus (corneoscleral junction).
Ask the patient to open and close his eyes to see whether
·ey close completely.

– If the downward movement of the upper eyelid in down gaze is delayed, the patient has a condition known as *lid la* (a common sign of hyperthyroidism).

- Assess the eyelids for redness, edema, inflammation, or lesions.

  – A stye, or *hordeolum*, is a common eyelid lesion.

- Watch for protrusion of the eyeball, called *exophthalmos* or *proptosis* (commonly occurs in patients with hyperthyroidism).

- Inspect the eyes for excessive tearing or dryness.

- Check the eyelid margins, which should be pink, and the eyelashes, which should turn outward.

- Observe whether the lower eyelids turn inward toward the eyeball (entropion) or outward (ectropion).

- Examine the eyelids for lumps.

- Palpate the nasolacrimal sac, following these steps:

  – Explain the procedure to the patient.

  – Put on examination gloves.

  – With the patient's eyes closed, gently palpate the area bel the inner canthus, noting tenderness, swelling, or discharg through the lacrimal point (which could indicate blockage the nasolacrimal duct).

Be sure to look for excessive tearing.

Conjunctiva

- Inspect the bulbar conjunctiva (the delicate mucous membrane that covers the exposed surface of the sclera).

  – Ask the patient to look up.

  – Gently pull down the lower eyelid.

Note excessive redness or exudate; the conjunctiva should
e clear and shiny.
Inspect for color changes, foreign bodies, and edema.
The sclera's color should be white to buff; in black patients,
ou may see flecks of tan (a bluish discoloration may indicate
cleral thinning).
xamine the palpebral conjunctiva (the membrane that lines
e eyelids), following these steps:
Ask the patient to look down.
Lift the upper lid, holding the upper lashes against the eye-
row with your finger.
The palpebral conjunctiva should be uniformly pink; in pa-
ents with a history of allergies, it may have a cobblestone ap-
earance.

rnea

xamine the cornea.
Shine a penlight first from both sides and then from straight
ead.
It should be clear and without lesions.
st corneal sensitivity.
Lightly touch the cornea with a wisp of cotton.

erior chamber

he anterior chamber should be bordered in the front by the
rnea and in the back by the iris.

he iris should appear flat.
he cornea should appear convex.
xcess pressure in the eye — such as that caused by acute an-
e-closure glaucoma — may push the iris forward, making
e anterior chamber appear very small.
th irises should be the same size, color, and shape.

Assessing corneal sensitivity

• Touch a wisp of cotton from a cotton ball to the cornea, as shown at right.
• The patient should blink. If he doesn't, he may have suffered damage to the sensory fibers of cranial nerve V or to the motor fibers controlled by cranial nerve VI.

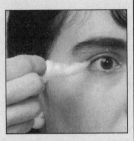

Keep in your mind's eye
• People who wear contact lenses may have reduced sensitivity because they're accustomed to having foreign objects in their eyes.
• A wisp of cotton is the only safe object to use for this test. Even though a 4″ × 4″ gauze pad or tissue is soft, it can cause corneal abrasions and irritation.

Pupil

• Each pupil should be equal in size to the other, round, and about one-fourth the size of the iris in normal room light.
    – Unequal pupils generally indicate neurologic damage, iritis glaucoma, or therapy with certain drugs.
    – About one person in four has asymmetrical pupils without disease.
    – A fixed pupil that doesn't react to light can be an ominous neurologic sign.
• Test the pupils for direct and consensual response.
    – In a slightly darkened room, hold a penlight about 20″ (50.8 cm) from the patient's eyes, and direct the light at the eye from the side.

Note the reaction of the pupil ou're testing (direct response) and the opposite pupil consensual response); both hould react the same way.

If you shine the light in a lind eye, neither pupil will espond.

Note sluggishness or inequaly in the response.

Repeat the test with the ther pupil.

est the pupils for accommoation.

Place your finger approxiately 4″ (10.2 cm) from the ridge of the patient's nose.

Ask the patient to look at a xed object in the distance and then to look at your finger; s pupils should constrict and his eyes converge as he focus- s on your finger.

> **Memory jogger**
>
> Here's a PERRLA of wisdom: To make sure that your pupil assessment is complete, think of the acronym PERRLA:
>
> Pupils
> Equal
> Round
> Reactive
> Light-responsive
> Accommodation.

ting visual acuity

llen chart

se the Snellen chart with a patient who can read.

Ask him to remove corrective lenses if he wears them.

Have the patient sit or stand 20′ (6.1 m) from the chart, and en cover his left eye with an opaque object.

Ask him to read the letters on one line of the chart and then move downward to increasingly smaller lines until he can longer discern all of the letters.

Have him repeat the test covering his right eye.

Have him read the smallest line he can read with both eyes covered to test his binocular vision.

– If the patient wears corrective lenses, have him repeat the test wearing them.
– Record his vision with and without correction.

- Use the Snellen E chart to test visual acuity in young children and other patients who can't read.
  – Cover the patient's left eye to check the right eye.
  – Point to an E on the chart.
  – Ask the patient to point which way the letter faces.
  – Repeat the test with the left eye.
- Suspect an eye abnormality, such as amblyopia, (especially in children) if the test values between the two eyes differ by two lines, for example, 20/30 in one eye and 20/50 in the other.

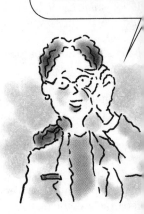

Patients who wear corrective lenses shou perform the Snellen chart test with and without the lenses.

Near-vision chart

- To test near vision:
  – Cover one of the patient's eyes with an opaque object.
  – Hold a Rosenbaum near-vision card 14″ (35.6 cm) from h eyes.
  – Have the patient read the line with the smallest letters he can distinguish.
  – Repeat the test with the other eye.
- If the patient wears corrective lenses, have him repeat the test while wearing them.
- Record the visual accommodation with and without lense

Visual acuity charts

The most commonly used charts for testing vision are the Snellen alphabet chart (below left) and the Snellen E chart (below right), the latter of which is used for young children and adults who can't read. Both charts are used to test distance vision and measure visual acuity. The patient reads each chart at a distance of 20' (6.1 m).

Recording results
• Record visual acuity as a fraction.
• The top number (20) is the distance between the patient and the chart.
• The bottom number is the distance from which a person with normal vision could read the line.
• The larger the bottom number, the poorer the patient's vision.

Age differences
• From age 6, normal vision is measured as 20/20.
• At age 5, normal vision is 20/30.
• At age 4, normal vision is 20/40.
• At age 3 and younger, normal vision is 20/50.

Snellen alphabet chart   **Snellen E chart**

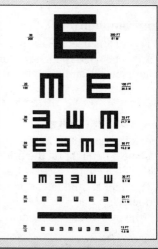

Using confrontation

- Sit directly across from the patient and have him focus his gaze on your eyes.
- Hold your hands about 2' (0.6 m) apart on either side of the patient's head at the level of his ears (as shown).
- Tell the patient to focus his gaze on you. Wiggle your fingers and gradually bring them into his visual field.
- Instruct the patient to tell you as soon as he can see your wiggling fingers, which should be at the same time you do.
- Repeat the procedure while holding your hands at the superior and inferior positions.

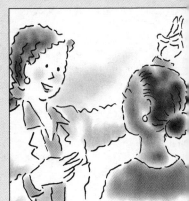

Confrontation

- This test is used to assess peripheral vision.
- It can be used to identify such abnormalities as homonymc hemianopia and bitemporal hemianopia.

Assessing eye muscle function

Corneal light reflex

- Ask the patient to look straight ahead.
- Shine a penlight on the bridge of his nose from about 12" to 15" (30.5 cm to 38 cm) away.
- The light should fall at the same spot on each cornea; if it doesn't:
  – the eyes aren't being held in the same plane by the extrac lar muscles

– the patient likely lacks muscle coordination, a condition called *strabismus.*

rdinal positions of gaze

This test helps evaluate:
- oculomotor, trigeminal, and abducent nerves
- extraocular muscles.

To perform the cardinal positions of gaze test:
- Ask the patient to remain still while you hold a pencil or other small object directly in front of his nose at a distance of about 18″ (45 cm).
- Ask him to follow the object with his eyes, without moving his head.
- Move the object to each of the six cardinal positions, returning to the midpoint after each movement.
- Note abnormal findings, such as nystagmus and amblyopia, which is the failure of one eye to follow an object (normally the patient's eyes remain parallel as they move).

Cardinal positions of gaze

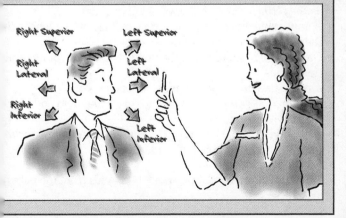

Cover-uncover test

- This test isn't done unless the corneal light reflex test and c dinal positions of gaze reveal an abnormality.
- To perform a cover-uncover test:
  - Have the patient stare at a wall on the other side of the room.
  - Cover one eye and watch for movement in the uncovered eye.
  - Remove the eye cover and watch for movement again.
  - Repeat the test with the other eye.
  - Note any eye movement while covering or uncovering the eye, which is considered abnormal (it may result from wea or paralyzed extraocular muscles, which may be caused by cranial nerve impairment).

Examining intraocular structures

- Use an ophthalmoscope to perform direct observation of tl eye's internal structures.
- Adjust the ophthalmoscope's lens disc.
- Use the green, positive numbers on the disc to focus on nea objects, such as the patient's cornea and lens.
- Use the red, minus numbers to focus on distant objects suc as the retina.
- If applicable, have the patient remove his contact lenses (if they're tinted) or eyeglasses.
- Darken the room to dilate the pupils and make your exami tion easier.
- Ask the patient to focus on a point behind you.
- Tell him that you'll be moving into his visual field and block ing his view.
- Explain that you'll be shining a bright light into his eye, wh may be uncomfortable but not harmful.
- Set the lens disc at zero.
- Hold the ophthalmoscope about 4″ (10 cm) from the patien eye.

Using an ophthalmoscope

This illustration shows the correct position for you and the patient when you use an ophthalmoscope to examine his eye's internal structures.

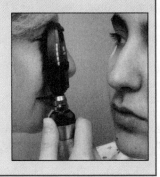

Direct the light through the pupil to elicit the red reflex (light reflecting off the choroids); check the red reflex for depth of color.

Move the ophthalmoscope closer to the eye.

Adjust the lens disc so you can focus on the anterior chamber and lens.

Look for clouding, foreign matter, or opacities; if the lens is opaque, indicating cataracts, you may not be able to complete the examination.

Turn the dial to zero to examine the retina.

Rotate the lens-power disc to adjust for your refractive correction and the patient's refractive error.

Observe the vitreous body for clarity; the first retinal structures you'll see are the blood vessels.

Rotate the dial into the negative numbers to bring the blood vessels into focus; the arteries will look thinner and brighter than the veins.

Follow one of the vessels along its path toward the nose until you reach the optic disk, where all vessels in the eye originate.

- Examine arteriovenous crossings for arteriovenous nicking (localized constrictions in the retinal vessels), which might be a sign of hypertension.
- Observe the optic disk, the creamy pink to yellow-orange structure with clear borders and a round-to-oval shape.
  – The optic disk may fill or exceed your field of vision.
  – If you don't see the optic disk, follow a blood vessel toward the center until you do.
- Identify the physiologic cup, which should occupy about one-third of the optic disk's diameter.
- Completely scan the retina by following four blood vessels from the optic disk to different peripheral areas; the retina should have a uniform color and be free from scars and pigmentation.
- Note any lesions or hemorrhages.
- Move the light laterally from the optic disk to locate the macula, the part of the eye most sensitive to light; it should appear as a darker structure that's free from blood vessels.

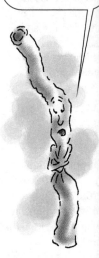

Constrictions in the retinal vessels may signal hypertension.

Abnormal findings

Amblyopia

Involves decreased vision in one eye because the brain favors the other eye
Sometimes referred to as *lazy eye*
Doesn't affect the eye's appearance
Ranks as the most common childhood vision impairment
Without treatment, persists into adulthood

Arteriolar narrowing

Involves narrowing of the arterioles
- Normally, appear to be about two-thirds to three-fourths the width of veins
- Appear about one-half as wide as veins when narrowed
Occurs in patients who have hypertension

Decreased visual acuity

Commonly occurs with refractive errors
Classified into two types
- Myopia (nearsightedness)—the eye focuses the visual image in front of the retina, causing objects in close view to be seen clearly and those at a distance to appear blurry
- Hyperopia (farsightedness)—the eye focuses the visual image behind the retina, causing objects in close view to appear blurry and those at a distance to seem clear

Diplopia

Also known as *double vision*
Involves misalignment of extraocular muscles; visual axes aren't directed at the object of sight at the same time, causing objects to appear twice

Discharge

Excretion of any substance from the eyes other than tears

Between the lines

Evaluating eye findings

Sign or symptom and findings	Probable cause
Eye discharge • Purulent or mucopurulent, greenish white discharge that occurs unilaterally • Sticky crusts that form on the eyelids during sleep • Itching and burning • Excessive tearing • Sensation of a foreign body in the eye	Bacterial conjunctiviti
• Scant but continuous purulent discharge that's easily expressed from the tear sac • Excessive tearing • Pain and tenderness near the tear sac • Eyelid inflammation and edema noticeable around the lacrimal punctum	Dacryocystitis
• Continuous frothy discharge • Chronically red eyes with inflamed lid margins • Soft, foul-smelling, cheesy yellow discharge elicited by pressure on the meibomian glands	Meibomianitis
Decreased visual acuity • Gradual visual blurring • Halo vision • Visual glare in bright light • Progressive vision loss • Gray pupil that later turns milky white	Cataract

Evaluating eye findings (continued)

Sign or symptom and findings	Probable cause
Decreased visual acuity (continued)	
Constant morning headache that decreases in severity during the day	Hypertension
Possible severe, throbbing headache	
Restlessness	
Confusion	
Nausea and vomiting	
Seizures	
Decreased level of consciousness	
Paroxysmal attacks of severe, throbbing unilateral or bilateral headache	Migraine headache
Nausea and vomiting	
Sensitivity to light and noise	
Sensory or visual auras	
Visual floaters	
Sudden onset of spots or flashing lights	Retinal detachment
Curtainlike loss of vision	
Black retinal vessels	
Onset of spots or flashing lights	Posterior uveitis
Gradual development of eye pain	
Photophobia	
Blurred vision	
Conjunctival injection	

■ May occur in one or both eyes
■ May be scant or copious
■ May be purulent, frothy, mucoid, cheesy, serous, or clear and have a stringy, white appearance

- Commonly results from inflammatory and infectious eye disorders such as conjunctivitis
- May occur in certain systemic disorders

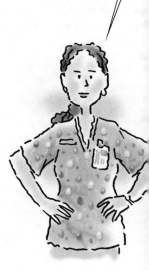

Eye pain requires immediate attention.

Pain

- May signal an emergency
- Requires immediate attention
- May be caused by:
  – acute angle-closure glaucoma
  – conjunctivitis
  – corneal damage caused by a foreign body or abrasion
  – trauma to the eye

Periorbital edema

- Swelling around the eyes
- May result from:
  – allergies
  – local inflammation
  – fluid-retaining disorders
  – crying

Ptosis

- Drooping upper eyelid
- May be caused by:
  – interruption in sympathetic innervation to the eyelid
  – muscle weakness
  – damage to the oculomotor nerve

Recognizing periorbital edema and ptosis

Periorbital edema

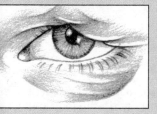

Ptosis

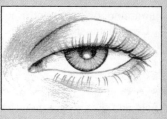

Strabismus

Deviation of the eyes from their normal gazing positions
Most commonly occurs in children
May result from:
- extraocular weakness or paralysis as a result of poor vision in one eye
- thyroid ophthalmopathy

Vision loss

May occur in various forms
- Central vision loss
- Peripheral vision loss
- Blind spot in the middle of an area of normal vision (scotoma)
Degree and location depends on:
- disease causing the problem
- location of the lesion
Can be caused by:
- glaucoma
- untreated cataracts

- retinal disease
- macular degeneration
- diabetic retinopathy
- opportunistic infections associated with HIV and acquired immunodeficiency syndrome
- toxoplasmosis
- cytomegalovirus retinitis

Visual floaters

- Specks of varying shape and size that float through the visual field and disappear when the patient tries to look at them
- Caused by small cells floating in the vitreous humor
- May signal:
  - vitreous hemorrhage
  - retinal separation
  - retinal detachment (if large and black)

Visual halos

- Seeing halos and rainbows around bright lights
- Caused by:
  - increased intraocular pressure (occurs in glaucoma)
  - corneal edema as a result of prolonged wearing of contact lenses or a fluctuation in blood glucose levels

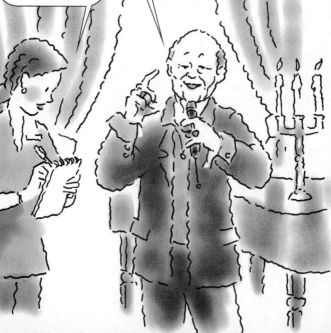

Health history

- Ask about the onset, location, duration, and characteristics symptoms.
- Ask what aggravates and relieves symptoms.

Asking about the ears

- Common ear complaints include:
  - hearing loss
  - tinnitus
  - pain
  - discharge
  - dizziness.

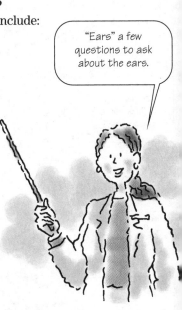

"Ears" a few questions to ask about the ears.

- Ask the patient about any associated symptoms.
- Have him describe the color and consistency of any ear discharge.
- Ask whether he has ever experienced a head injury.
- Ask about any feelings of abnormal movement or vertigo (spinning) and determine:
  - when the episodes occur
  - how frequently they occur
  - whether they're associated with nausea, vomiting, or tinnitus.
- Ask about previous ear problems or injury.
- Ask whether anyone in the patient's family has ear or hearing problems.
- Ask whether the patient has recently been ill or has a chronic disorder.

- Diabetes can cause hearing loss.
- Hypertension can cause high-pitched tinnitus.

Ask about current treatments and medications.
- Certain antibiotics and other medications can cause hearing loss and tinnitus.

Ask whether the patient has allergies or a history of inflammation of the middle or external ear.
- *Serous otitis media* (inflammation of the middle ear) is common in people with environmental or seasonal allergies.
- *Otitis externa* (inflammation of the external ear) can be caused by allergic reactions to hair dyes, cosmetics, perfumes, and other personal care products.

king about the nose

Common complaints about the nose include:
- nasal stuffiness
- nasal discharge
- epistaxis (nosebleed).

Ask the patient whether he has frequent colds, hay fever, headaches, or sinus trouble.
Determine whether certain conditions or places seem to cause or aggravate the patient's problem.
Ask whether he has ever had nose or head trauma.
Inquire about the color and consistency of nasal discharge.

king about the mouth, throat, and neck

Ask the patient about:
- bleeding or sore gums
- mouth or tongue ulcers
- bad taste in the mouth
- bad breath
- toothaches or loose teeth
- frequent sore throats
- hoarseness
- facial swelling.

- Ask whether the patient smokes or uses other types of tobacco.
- Ask whether he has:
  - neck pain or tenderness
  - neck swelling
  - trouble moving his neck.

Asking about general health

- Ask the patient about his general health.
- Be alert for responses that might indicate a thyroid disorde
  - Hyperthyroidism can cause heat intolerance and weight loss. Women with hyperthyroidism may have a short menst al pattern with scant flow.
  - Hypothyroidism can cause cold intolerance, weight gain and, in extreme cases, bradycardia and dyspnea from low c diac output. Women may experience increased frequency a flow of menses.
- Ask the patient these questions pertaining to signs and sym toms:
  - Have you noticed changes in the way you tolerate hot and cold weather?
  - Has your weight changed recently?
  - Do you have breathing problems or feel as if your heart is skipping beats?
  - Have you noticed any tremors, agitation, or difficulty con- centrating or sleeping?
  - Have you noticed a change in your menstrual pattern?

Physical assessment

Examining the ears, nose, and throat mainly involves using the techniques of inspection, palpation, and auscultation. Ear assessment also requires:
- use of an otoscope
- administration of hearing acuity tests.

Examining the ears

External observations

Observe the ears for position and symmetry.
- The top of the ear should line up with the outer corner of the eye.
- Both ears should look symmetrical, with an angle of attachment of no more than 10 degrees.
- The face and ears should be the same shade and color.
- Auricles that protrude from the head are fairly common and don't affect hearing ability.
- Low-set ears commonly accompany congenital disorders, including kidney problems.

Inspect the auricle for lesions, drainage, nodules, or redness.

Pull the helix back and ask the patient about tenderness. If pulling the ear back hurts, he may have otitis externa. Note your findings.

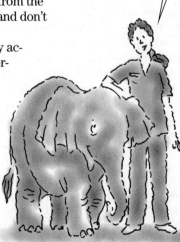

No matter what size the patient's ears are, you should observe their position and symmetry.

- Inspect and palpate the mastoid area behind each auricle, noting tenderness, redness, or warmth.
- Inspect the opening of the ear canal, noting discharge, redness, odor, or the presence of nodules or cysts.
  – Hair and *cerumen* (earwax) normally appear in the ear canal; the amount of each varies.

Otoscopic examination

- Examine the auditory canal, tympanic membrane, and malle
- Check the canal for foreign bodies or discharge before inse ing the speculum into the ear canal.
- Palpate the tragus (the cartilaginous projection anterior to the external opening of the ear) and pull the auricle up. If th area is tender, don't insert the speculum; otitis externa may be present, and inserting the speculum could be painful.
- To insert the speculum of the otoscope:
  – Tilt the patient's head away from you.
  – Grasp the superior posterior auricle with your thumb and dex finger, and pull it up and back to straighten the canal.
  – Vary the angle of the speculum until you can see the tympanic membrane. If the patient is younger than age 3, pull th auricle down to get a good view.
  – Hold the otoscope with one hand and brace your hand against the patient's head for steadiness.
  – Insert the speculum gently into the ear canal (the inner tw thirds of the canal is sensitive to pressure), directing it dow and forward. Inspect the ear canal.
- Note the cerumen color and consistency. Be aware that eld ly patients may have harder, drier cerumen.
- The external canal should be free from inflammation and scaling.
- If the view of the tympanic membrane is obstructed by exce sive cerumen:
  – don't try to remove the cerumen with an instrument.
  – use ceruminolytic drops and warm water irrigation as ordered.

Help desk

Using an otoscope

Inserting the speculum

Before inserting the speculum into the patient's ear, straighten the ear canal by grasping the auricle and pulling it up and back.

Positioning the scope

To examine the ear's external canal, hold the otoscope with the handle parallel to the patient's head, as shown below.

Brace your hand firmly against his head to avoid cutting the canal with the speculum.

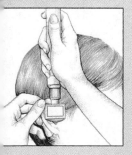

Viewing the structures

• When the otoscope is positioned properly, you should see the tympanic membrane structures shown below.

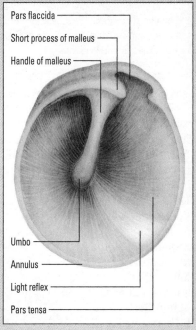

Pars flaccida

Short process of malleus

Handle of malleus

Umbo

Annulus

Light reflex

Pars tensa

• You may need to carefully rotate the speculum for a complete view of the tympanic membrane.

• The tympanic membrane should be a pearl-gray color, glistening, and transparent.

Different strokes

Cerumen variations

When examining your patient's ear canal, keep in mind that the presence of cerumen doesn't indicate poor hygiene. In fact, the appearance and type of cerumen is genetically determined. There are two types of cerumen:
• dry cerumen — gray and flaky; mostly found in Asians and Native Americans (including Eskimos)
• wet cerumen — dark brown and moist; commonly found in Blacks and Whites.

– The annulus (the ring-shaped structure around the tympanic membrane) should be white and denser than the rest of the tympanic membrane.
• Inspect the tympanic membrane carefully for bulging, retraction, bleeding, lesions, and perforations, especially at the periphery.
• Keep in mind that an elderly patient's tympanic membranes may appear cloudy.
• Examine the tympanic membrane for the light reflex.
  – In the right ear, the light reflex should be between 4 and 6 o'clock.
  – In the left ear, the light reflex should be between 6 and 8 o'clock.

An older patient's tympanic membrane may appear cloudy.

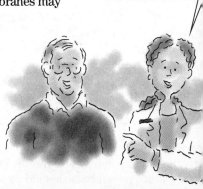

Absent or displaced light indicates that the tympanic membrane may be bulging, inflamed, or retracted.

Look for the bony landmarks.

The malleus will appear as a dense, white streak at the 2 o'clock position.

The umbo (inferior point of the malleus) will appear at the top of the light reflex.

Hearing acuity tests

Weber's test and the Rinne test are used to assess:

conduction hearing loss

impaired sound transmission to the inner ear

sensorineural hearing loss

impaired auditory nerve conduction or inner ear function.

Weber's test

Perform Weber's test when the patient reports diminished or lost hearing in one ear.

In this test, a tuning fork is used to evaluate bone conduction. The tuning fork should be tuned to the frequency of normal human speech, 512 cycles/second.

To perform Weber's test:

Strike the tuning fork lightly against your hand.

Place the fork on the patient's forehead at the midline or on the top of his head.

The test is normal if the tone is heard equally well in both ears.

If the tone is heard better in one ear, record the result as right or left lateralization.

If the tone is heard in the patient's impaired ear, he has conductive hearing loss.

If the tone is heard in his unaffected ear, he has sensorineural hearing loss.

Rinne test

Perform the Rinne test after Weber's test to compare air conduction of sound with bone conduction of sound.

- To administer the Rinne test:
  – Strike the tuning fork against your hand.
  – Place the tuning fork over the patient's mastoid process.
  – Ask him to tell you when the tone stops; note the length o
  time in seconds.
  – Move the still-vibrating tuning fork to the ear's opening w
  out touching the ear.

Help desk

Positioning the tuning fork

Weber's test
- With the tuning fork vibrating lightly, position the tip on the patient's forehead at the midline.
- Alternatively, place the tuning fork on the top of the patient's head, as shown.

Rinne test
- Strike the tuning fork against your hand, and then hold it behir the patient's ear, as shown.
- When your patient tells you the tone has stopped, move the still-vibrating tuning fork to the opening of his ear.

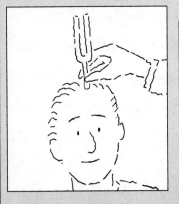

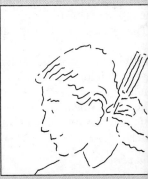

Physical assessment **109**

> Ask him to tell you when the tone stops; note the time in seconds.
> The test is normal if the air-conducted tone is heard twice as long as the bone-conducted tone.
> If the bone-conducted tone is heard as long as or longer than the air-conducted tone, conductive hearing loss is present.
> If the air-conducted sound is heard longer than the bone-conducted sound, sensorineural hearing loss is present.

Examining the nose and sinuses

Inspecting and palpating the nose

> Observe the patient's nose for position, symmetry, and color.
> Note variations, such as discoloration, swelling, or deformity.
> Check for variations in size and shape, which are largely caused by differences in cartilage and in the amount of fibro-adipose tissue.
> Observe for nasal discharge or flaring.
> If discharge is present, note the color, quantity, and consistency.
> If flaring is noted, observe for other signs of respiratory distress.
> Test nasal patency and olfactory nerve (cranial nerve I) function.
> Ask the patient to block one nostril and inhale a familiar aromatic substance (soap, coffee, citrus, tobacco, or nutmeg) through the other nostril.
> Ask him to identify the aroma.
> Repeat the process with the other nostril, using a different aroma.
> Inspect the nasal cavity.
> Ask the patient to tilt his head back slightly, and then push the tip of his nose up.
> Use the light from the otoscope to illuminate his nasal cavities.

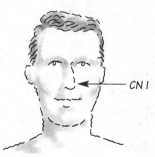

CN I

– Check for severe deviation or perforation of the nasal septum.

– Examine the vestibule and turbinates for redness, softnes swelling, and discharge.

- Examine the nostrils by direct inspection.

- Use a nasal speculum, a penlight or small flashlight, or an oto-scope with a short, wide-tip attachment.

- Have the patient sit in front of you with his head tilted back.

- Put on gloves and in-sert the tip of the closed nasal speculum into one nostril to the point where the blade widens.

- Slowly open the speculum as wide as possible without causing discomfort.

- Shine the flashlight in the nostril to illuminate the area.

- Observe the color and patency of the nostril, and check f exudate (the mucosa should be moist, pink to light red, an free from lesions and polyps).

- After inspecting one nostril, close the speculum, remove and inspect the other nostril.

- Palpate the patient's nose with your thumb and forefinger, sessing for pain, tenderness, swelling, and deformity.

Examining the sinuses

- Examine the sinuses.

- Only the frontal and maxillary sinuses are accessible; you won't be able to palpate the ethmoidal and sphenoidal sinuses.

Inspecting the nostrils

The illustration at right shows the proper placement of the nasal speculum during direct inspection and the structures you should be able to see during this examination.

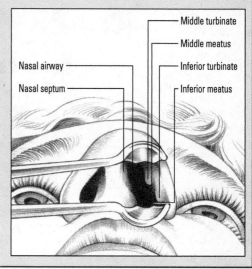

Nasal airway

Nasal septum

Middle turbinate

Middle meatus

Inferior turbinate

Inferior meatus

If the frontal and maxillary sinuses are infected, you can assume that the other sinuses are also.
▶ Check for swelling around the eyes, especially over the sinus area.
▶ Palpate the sinuses, checking for tenderness.
▶ To palpate the frontal sinuses:
– Place your thumbs above the patient's eyes just under the bony ridges of the upper orbits, and place your fingertips on his forehead.
– Apply gentle pressure.
▶ To palpate the maxillary sinuses:
– Place your thumbs on each side of the nose just below the cheekbones, and place your fingertips on his forehead.
– Apply gentle pressure.

Palpating the maxillary sinuses

Gently press your thumbs on each side of the nose just below the cheekbones, as shown. Tenderness may indicate that the sinuses are infected. Note also the location of the frontal sinuses, for palpation.

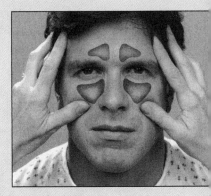

Examining the mouth, throat, and neck

Assessing the mouth and throat

- Inspect the patient's lips.
  - They should be pink, moist, symmetrical, and without lesions.
  - A bluish hue or flecked pigmentation is common in dark-skinned patients.
- Put on gloves and palpate the lips for lumps or surface abnormalities.
- Use a tongue blade and a bright light to inspect the oral mucosa.
  - Have the patient open his mouth.
  - Place the tongue blade on top of his tongue.
  - The oral mucosa should be pink, smooth, moist, and free from lesions and unusual odors; increased pigmentation is common in dark-skinned patients.
- Observe the gingivae, or gums.
  - They should be pink and moist and have clearly defined margins at each tooth.

They shouldn't be retracted.

Inspect the teeth.

Note their number, their condition, and whether any are missing or crowded.

If the patient is wearing dentures, ask him to remove them so you can inspect the gums underneath.

Inspect the tongue.

It should be midline, moist, pink, and free from lesions.

The posterior surface should be smooth.

The anterior surface should be slightly rough with small fissures.

The tongue should move easily in all directions, and it should lie straight to the front at rest.

Ask the patient to raise the tip of his tongue and touch his palate directly behind his front teeth.

Inspect the ventral surface of the tongue and the floor of the mouth.

Wrap a piece of gauze around the tip of the tongue and move the tongue first to one side then the other to inspect the lateral borders (they should be smooth and even-textured).

Inspect the patient's oropharynx.

Ask him to open his mouth while you shine the penlight on the uvula and palate.

You may need to insert a tongue blade into the mouth and depress the tongue.

Place the tongue blade slightly off center to avoid eliciting the gag reflex.

The uvula and oropharynx should be pink and moist, without inflammation or exudate.

The tonsils should be pink and shouldn't be hypertrophied (enlarged).

Ask the patient to say "Ahhh" while you observe the movement of the soft palate and uvula.

Palpate the lips, tongue, and oropharynx.

Note lumps, lesions, ulcers, or edema of the lips or tongue.

Assess the patient's gag reflex.

– Gently touch the back of the pharynx with a cotton-tipped
applicator or the tongue blade; this should produce a bilateral
response.

Inspecting and palpating the neck

- Observe the patient's neck.
  – It should be symmetrical, and the skin should be intact.
  – Note any scars.
  – No visible pulsations, masses, swelling, venous distention,
  or thyroid or lymph node enlargement should be present.
  – Ask the patient to move his neck through the entire range
  motion and to shrug his shoulders.
  – Ask him to swallow, and note rising of the larynx, trachea,
  or thyroid.
- Palpate the patient's neck.
  – Using the finger pads of both hands, bilaterally palpate the
  chain of lymph nodes under the patient's chin in the preauric-
  ular area.
  – Proceed to the area under and behind the ears.
  – Assess the nodes for size, shape, mobility, consistency, tem-
  perature, and tenderness, comparing nodes on one side with
  those on the other.
- Palpate the trachea (normally located midline in the neck).
  – Place your thumbs along each side of the trachea near the
  lower part of the neck.
  – Assess whether the distance between the trachea's outer
  edge and the sternocleidomastoid muscle is equal on both
  sides.
- Palpate the thyroid.
  – Stand behind the patient and put your hands around his
  neck, with the fingers of both hands over the lower trachea.
  – Ask him to swallow as you feel the thyroid isthmus.
  – The isthmus should rise with swallowing because it lies
  across the trachea, just below the cricoid cartilage.

ymph node locations

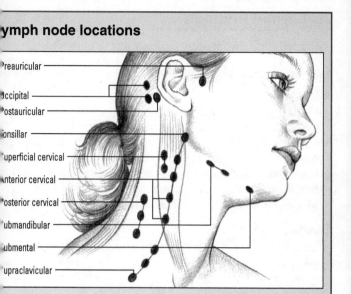

- Preauricular
- Occipital
- Postauricular
- Tonsillar
- Superficial cervical
- Anterior cervical
- Posterior cervical
- Submandibular
- Submental
- Supraclavicular

Displace the thyroid to the right and then to the left, palpating both lobes for enlargement, nodules, tenderness, or a gritty sensation.

Auscultating the neck

Using light pressure on the bell of the stethoscope, listen over the carotid arteries.

Ask the patient to hold his breath while you listen; this prevents breath sounds from interfering with the sounds of circulation.

Listen for bruits, which signal turbulent blood flow.

Auscultate the thyroid area with the bell if you detect an enlarged thyroid gland.

Check for a bruit or a soft rushing sound, which indicates a hypermetabolic state.

Abnormal findings

- Record your findings and evaluate any abnormalities.

Ear abnormalities

Earache

- Usually results from disorders of the external and middle ear associated with infection, obstruction, or trauma
- Ranges in severity from a feeling of fullness or blockage to a deep, penetrating pain
- May be difficult to determine precise location of an earache
- Can be intermittent or continuous
- May develop suddenly or gradually

Hearing loss

- If onset is rapid, may result from a toxic reaction to drugs, such as:
  - aspirin
  - aminoglycosides
  - loop diuretics
  - certain chemotherapeutic agents, including cisplatin
- Conductive hearing loss caused by:
  - ear canal obstruction from cerumen, foreign body, or polyp
  - thickened fluid in the middle ear, resulting from otitis media, which interferes with the vibrations that transmit sound
  - otosclerosis, a hardening of the bones in the middle ear, which interferes with the transmission of sound vibrations
  - Trauma that disrupts the middle ear's bony chain
- Sensorineural hearing loss caused by:
  - Loss of hair cells in the organ of Corti
  - Atrophy of the organ of Corti and the auditory nerve (progressive hearing loss is common in elderly patients)
  - Trauma to the hair cells caused by loud noise or ototoxicity

Otorrhea

- Drainage from the ear

(Text continues on page)

Between the lines

Evaluating ear, nose, and throat findings

Signs or symptom and findings	Probable cause
Dysphagia	
Signs of respiratory distress, such as crowing and stridor	Airway obstruction
Phase 2 dysphagia with gagging and dysphonia	
Phase 2 and 3 dysphagia	Esophageal cancer
Rapid weight loss	
Steady chest pain	
Cough with hemoptysis	
Hoarseness	
Sore throat	
Hiccups	
Painless, progressive dysphagia	Lead poisoning
Lead line on the gums	
Metallic taste	
Papilledema	
Ocular palsy	
Footdrop or wristdrop	
Mental impairment or seizures	
Earache	
Sensation of blockage or fullness in the ear	Cerumen impaction
Itching	
Partial hearing loss	
Possible dizziness	

(continued)

Evaluating ear, nose, and throat findings *(continued)*

Signs or symptom and findings	Probable cause
Earache *(continued)* • Mild to moderate ear pain that occurs with tragus manipulation • Low-grade fever • Sticky yellow or purulent ear discharge • Partial hearing loss • Feeling of blockage in the ear • Swelling of the tragus, external meatus, and external canal • Lymphadenopathy	Otitis externa
• Severe, deep, throbbing pain • Hearing loss • High fever • Bulging, fiery red eardrum	Acute otitis med
Epistaxis • Ecchymoses • Petechiae • Bleeding from gums, mouth, and I.V. puncture sites • Menorrhagia • Signs of GI bleeding, such as melena and hematemesis	Coagulation disorders
• Unilateral or bilateral epistaxis • Nasal swelling • Periorbital ecchymoses and edema • Pain • Nasal deformity • Crepitation of the nasal bones	Nasal fracture

valuating ear, nose, and throat findings *(continued)*

gns or symptom and findings	Probable cause
pistaxis *(continued)*	
Oozing epistaxis	Typhoid fever
Dry cough	
Abrupt onset of chills and high fever	
"Rose-spot" rash	
Vomiting	
Profound fatigue	
Anorexia	
asal obstruction	
Watery nasal discharge	Common cold
Sneezing	
Temporary loss of smell and taste	
Sore throat	
Malaise	
Arthralgia	
Mild headache	
Anosmia	Nasal polyps
Clear, watery nasal discharge	
History of allergies, chronic sinusitis, trauma, ystic fibrosis, or asthma	
Translucent, pear-shaped polyps that are unilateral or bilateral	
Thick, purulent drainage	Sinusitis
Severe pain over the sinuses	
Fever	
Inflamed nasal mucosa with purulent mucus	

(continued)

Evaluating ear, nose, and throat findings (continued)

Signs or symptom and findings	Probable cause
Throat pain	
• Throat pain that occurs seasonally or year-round	Allergic rhinitis
• Nasal congestion with a thin nasal discharge and postnasal drip	
• Paroxysmal sneezing	
• Decreased sense of smell	
• Frontal or temporal headache	
• Pale and glistening nasal mucosa with edematous nasal turbinates	
• Watery eyes	Laryngitis
• Mild to severe hoarseness	
• Temporary loss of voice	
• Malaise	
• Low-grade fever	
• Dysphagia	
• Dry cough	
• Tender, enlarged cervical lymph nodes	
• Mild to severe sore throat	Tonsillitis, acute
• Pain may radiate to the ears	
• Dysphagia	
• Headache	
• Malaise	
• Fever with chills	
• Tender cervical lymphadenopathy	

- May be bloody (otorrhagia), purulent, clear, or serosanguineous
- May occur alone or with other symptoms such as ear pain
- May be of varying onset, duration, and severity (can provid clues about the underlying cause)

May result from disorders that affect the external ear canal or the middle ear, including:
- allergies
- infection
- neoplasms
- trauma
- collagen disease

Nose, mouth, and throat abnormalities

Epistaxis
Also referred to as a *nosebleed*
Can occur spontaneously or be induced from the front or back of the nose
May be triggered by:
- dry, irritated mucous membranes that are more susceptible to infection
- trauma
- septal deviation
- hematologic, coagulation, renal, and GI disorders
- certain drugs and treatments

Nasal flaring
Can occur normally during quiet breathing in adults and children
May signal respiratory distress in an adult if marked and regular

Nasal stuffiness and discharge
Mucous membrane obstruction and discharge of thin mucus indicates:
- systemic disorders
- nasal or sinus disorders, such as a deviated septum
- trauma, such as a basilar skull or nasal fracture
- excessive use of vasoconstricting nose drops or sprays
- allergies or exposure to irritants, such as dust, tobacco smoke, and fumes.

- Nasal drainage accompanied by sinus tenderness and fever indicates acute sinusitis, which usually involves the frontal maxillary sinuses.
- Thick, white, yellow, or greenish drainage suggests infection
- Clear, thin drainage may be cerebrospinal fluid leaking from basilar skull fracture or other defect.

Dysphagia

- Refers to difficulty swallowing
- Most common symptom of esophageal disorders
- May result from:
  – oropharyngeal, respiratory, neurologic, and collagen disorders
  – toxins
  – treatments
- Increases the risk of choking and aspiration

Throat pain

- Commonly known as a *sore throat*
- Refers to discomfort in any part of the pharynx
- Ranges from a sensation of scratchiness to severe pain
- May result from:
  – infection
  – trauma
  – allergies
  – cancer
  – systemic disorders
  – surgery or endotracheal intubation
  – mouth breathing
  – alcohol consumption
  – inhaling smoke or chemicals such as ammonia
  – vocal strain

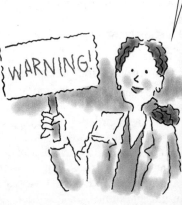

Dysphagia increases the risk of choking and aspiration.

WARNING!

Respiratory system

8

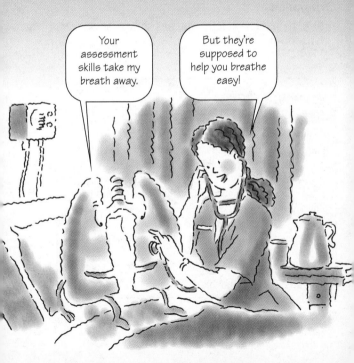

Health history

Asking about the respiratory system

Shortness of breath

- Ask the patient to rate his usual level of dyspnea on a scale 0 to 10; then ask him to rate his level that day.
  - Rating of 0 means no dyspnea.
  - Rating of 10 means the worst he has experienced.
- Other scales grade dyspnea as it relates to activity.
- Also ask these questions:
  - What do you do to relieve your difficulty breathing?
  - How well do relief measures work?

Orthopnea

- Ask the patient whether he has shortness of breath when lying down.

Grading dyspnea

- *Grade 0:* not troubled by breathlessness except with strenuous exercise
- *Grade 1:* troubled by shortness of breath when hurrying on a level path or walking up a slight hill
- *Grade 2:* walks more slowly on a level path than people of the same age because of breathlessness or has to stop to breathe when walking on a level path at his own pace
- *Grade 3:* stops to breathe after walking about 100 yards (91 m) on a level path
- *Grade 4:* too breathless to leave the house or breathless when dressing or undressing

Ask whether he tends to sleep with his upper body elevated.
Ask the patient how many pillows he uses.
- A patient who uses three pillows can be said to have three-pillow orthopnea."

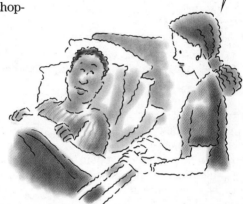

You must have a pretty tough time breathing when you're lying down.

Cough

Ask these questions about a patient's cough:
- Is the cough productive?
- If the cough is a chronic problem, has it changed recently? If so, how?
- What makes the cough better?
- What makes the cough worse?

Sputum

Ask the patient to estimate the amount of sputum, or mucus, produced in teaspoons or another common measurement. Also ask these questions about sputum production:
- At what time of day does sputum production most often occur?
- What are the color and consistency of the sputum?
- If sputum is a chronic problem, has it changed recently? If so, how?
- Is the sputum ever accompanied by blood? If so, how much and how often does this occur?

Wheezing

- Ask these questions about wheezing:
  - When does the wheezing occur?
  - What causes the wheezing?
  - Do others hear the wheezing?
  - What helps stop the wheezing?

Chest pain

- Ask these questions about chest pain:
  - Where's the pain?
  - What does it feel like? Is it sharp, stabbing, burning, or aching?
  - Does it move to another area?
  - How long does it last?
  - What triggers it?
  - What makes it better?
- Keep in mind that chest pain associated with respiratory problems is usually caused by pneumonia, pulmonary embolism, or pleural inflammation.
- Also keep in mind that coughing or fractures can cause musculoskeletal chest pain.

Questions about general health

- Look at the patient's medical and family history, particularly
  - smoking habits
  - allergies
  - previous operations
  - respiratory diseases, such as pneumonia and tuberculosis.
- Ask about environmental or occupational exposure to irritants such as asbestos.

Physical assessment

Use a systematic approach to detect subtle or obvious respiratory changes.
Physical examination of the respiratory system requires:
- inspection
- palpation
- percussion
- auscultation.

Take a few observations as you enter the patient's room.
- How is the patient seated?
- What is his awareness level?
- Does he appear relaxed?
- Does he appear anxious?
- Does he appear uncomfortable?
- Is he having trouble breathing?

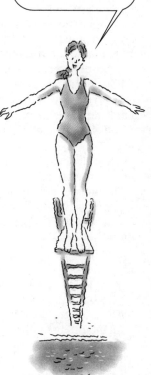

Take a deep breath. We're about to dive into respiratory assessment!

Memory jogger

To remember the order in which you should perform assessment of most body systems, just think, I'll **P**roperly **P**erform **A**ssessment:

Inspection

Palpation

Percussion

Auscultation.

Inspecting the chest

- Introduce yourself and explain why you're there.
- Help the patient into an upright position.
- Have the patient undress from the waist up or put on an examination gown that allows access to the chest.
- Examine the back of the chest first.
  - Use inspection, palpation, percussion, and auscultation.
  - Compare one side with the other.
- Examine the front of the chest using the same sequence.
- Note masses or scars that indicate surgery or trauma.
- Look for chest wall symmetry.
  - Both sides of the chest should be equal at rest and should expand equally as the patient inhales.
- Look at the diameter of the chest, from front to back.
  - The chest diameter should be about half the width of the chest.
- Look at the costal angle (angle between the ribs and the sternum at the point immediately above the xiphoid process).
  - The angle should be less than 90 degrees in an adult.
  - The angle will be larger if the chest wall is chronically expanded, as can happen with chronic obstructive pulmonary disease (COPD).
- Count the patient's respiratory rate for a full minute — long if you note abnormalities.
  - Don't tell the patient what you're doing because he might ter his breathing pattern.
  - Adults normally breathe at a rate of 12 to 20 breaths/minu
  - An infant's breathing rate may reach about 40 breaths/minute.
- The respiratory pattern should be even, coordinated, and r ular, with occasional sighs.
- The appropriate ratio of inspiration to expiration (I:E) is about 1:2.
- Watch for paradoxical, or uneven, movement of the chest wall, indicating loss of normal chest wall function, such as:

- abnormal collapse of part of the chest wall when the patient inhales
- abnormal expansion when the patient exhales.

The abdomen should push out and the lower ribs should expand laterally during inhalation.

The abdomen and ribs should return to their resting positions during exhalation.

Frequent use of accessory muscles may be normal in some athletes; however, for other patients, it indicates a respiratory problem, particularly when the patient purses his lips and flares his nostrils when breathing.

Inspecting related structures

A bluish tint to the skin and mucous membranes indicates cyanosis.

- Cyanosis occurs when oxygenation to the tissues is poor.
- It's a late sign of hypoxemia.
- The tongue and mucous membranes of the mouth are the most reliable places to check for cyanosis.

Check the fingers for clubbing, a possible sign of long-term hypoxia.

- Fingernails normally enter the skin at an angle of less than 180 degrees.
- When clubbing occurs, the angle is greater than or equal to 180 degrees.

Palpating the chest

Palpate gently.

The chest wall should feel smooth, warm, and dry.

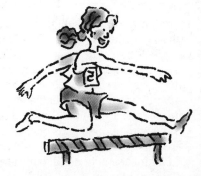

Use of accessory muscles may be normal in some athletes.

Palpating the chest

- Place the palm of your hand (or hands) lightly over the thorax, as shown below left.
- Palpate for tenderness, alignment, bulging, and retractions of the chest and intercostal spaces.
- Assess the patient for crepitus, especially around drainage sites. Repeat this procedure on the patient's back.

- Use the pads of your fingers, as shown below right, to palpate the front and back of the thorax.
- Pass your fingers over the ribs and any scars, lumps, lesions, or ulcerations.
- Note the skin temperature, turgor, and moisture.
- Also note tenderness and bony or subcutaneous crepitus.

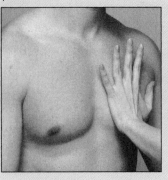
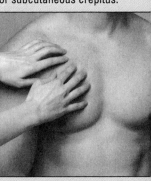

- Crepitus indicates subcutaneous air in the chest from leaking airways or lungs—an abnormal condition.
  – It feels like puffed-rice cereal crackling under the skin.
  – A small amount of subcutaneous air may be found around the insertion site of a patient's chest tube.
  – Notify the doctor immediately if the patient has no chest tube or the area of crepitus is getting larger.
- If the patient complains of chest pain, try to find a painful area on the chest wall.
  – Painful costochondral joints are typically located at the m clavicular line or next to the sternum.

- Areas over rib or vertebral fractures are typically quite painful; pain may also radiate around the chest.
- Pain may also result from sore muscles caused by protracted coughing or a collapsed lung.

Palpate for *tactile fremitus*, palpable vibrations caused by the transmission of air through the bronchopulmonary system. Tactile fremitus is decreased:
- over areas where pleural fluid collects
- at times when the patient speaks softly
- with pneumothorax, atelectasis, and emphysema.

Increased tactile fremitus is normal over the large bronchial tubes.

Increased tactile fremitus is abnormal over areas where alveoli are filled with fluid or exudate (as happens in pneumonia).

Checking for tactile fremitus

Ask the patient to fold his arms cross his chest. This movement shifts the scapulae out of the way.

Check for tactile fremitus by lightly placing your open palms on both sides of the patient's back, as shown at right, without touching his back with your fingers.

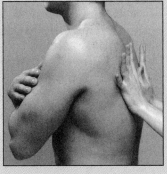

Ask the patient to repeat the phrase "ninety-nine" loud enough to produce palpable vibrations.

Palpate the front of the chest using the same hand positions.

Vibrations that feel more intense on one side than the other indicate tissue consolidation on that side.

Less intense vibrations may indicate emphysema, pneumothorax, or pleural effusion.

Faint or no vibrations in the upper posterior thorax may indicate bronchial obstruction or a fluid-filled pleural space.

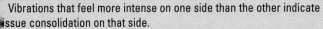

- Evaluate chest wall symmetry and expansion.
  – Place your hands on the front of the chest wall with your thumbs touching each other at the second intercostal space
  – As the patient inhales deeply, watch your thumbs; they should separate simultaneously to an equal distance several centimeters away from the sternum.
  – Repeat the measurement at the fifth intercostal space; tak the same measurement on the back of the chest near the ter rib.
  – The patient's chest may expand asymmetrically if he has pleural effusion, atelectasis, pneumonia, or pneumothorax.
  – Expansion may lessen at the level of the diaphragm if the patient has emphysema, respiratory depression, diaphragm paralysis, atelectasis, obesity, or ascites.

Percussing the chest

- Percuss the chest to determine:
  – lung boundaries
  – whether the lungs are filled with air, fluid, or solid materia
  – the distance the diaphragm travels between the patient's in halation and exhalation.
- Percussion allows you to assess structures as deep as $3''$ (7.6 cm).
- Different percussion sounds are heard in different areas of the chest.
  – Resonant sounds are heard over normal lung tissue, which you should find over most of the chest.
  – You should hear a dull sound over the space occupied by t heart (the left front chest from the third or fourth intercosta space at the sternum to the third or fourth intercostal space the midclavicular line).
  – Resonance resumes at the sixth intercostal space.
- The sequence of sounds in the back is slightly different from the front.
- Hyperresonance during percussion:

Percussing the chest

If you're right-handed, hyperextend the middle finger of your left hand; if you're left-handed, hyperextend the middle finger of your right hand.

Place this hand firmly on the patient's chest.

With the tip of the middle finger of your dominant hand, tap on the middle finger of your other hand just below the distal joint (as shown).

Follow the standard percussion sequence over the front and back chest walls.

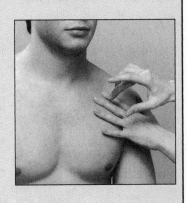

- indicates an area of increased air in the lung or pleural space
- occurs with pneumothorax, acute asthma, bullous emphysema (large holes in the lungs from alveolar destruction), or gastric distention that pushes up on the diaphragm.

Abnormal dullness:
- indicates areas of decreased air in the lungs
- occurs in the presence of pleural fluid, consolidation, atelectasis, or a tumor.

You may hear different sounds after certain treatments, such as chest physiotherapy.

Use other assessment techniques to confirm percussion findings.

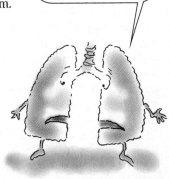

Hyperresonance indicates increased air in the lung or pleural space.

Percussion sequences

Follow these percussion sequences to distinguish between normal and abnormal sounds in the patient's lungs. Compare sound variations from one side with the other as you proceed. Carefully describe abnormal sounds you hear and include their locations. You'll follow the same sequences for auscultation.

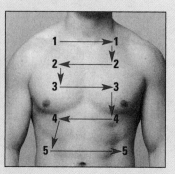
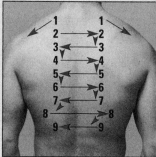

Auscultating the chest

- Air moves through the bronchi creating sound waves that travel to the chest wall.
- Sounds change:
  – as air moves from larger airways to smaller airways.
  – if air passes through fluid, mucus, or narrowed airways.
- Auscultation helps you determine the condition of the alveo and surrounding pleura.
- Auscultation sites are the same as percussion sites.
- Listen to a full inspiration and a full expiration at each site, using the diaphragm of the stethoscope.
- Ask the patient to breathe through his mouth; nose breathin alters the pitch of breath sounds.
- If the patient has abundant chest hair, dampen it with a was cloth so the hair doesn't make sounds that could be confuse with crackles.

Between the lines

Percussion sounds

Sound	Description	Clinical significance
Flat	Short, soft, high-pitched, extremely dull	Consolidation, as in atelectasis and extensive pleural effusion
Dull	Medium in intensity and pitch, moderate length, thudlike	Solid area, as in lobar pneumonia
Resonant	Long, loud, low-pitched, hollow	Normal lung tissue; bronchitis
Hyperresonant	Very loud, lower-pitched	Hyperinflated lung, as in emphysema or pneumothorax
Tympanic	Loud, high-pitched, moderate length, musical, drumlike	Air collection, as in a gastric air bubble, air in the intestines, or a large pneumothorax

Press the stethoscope firmly against the skin.

You'll hear four types of breath sounds over normal lungs:
- Tracheal breath sounds—heard above the supraclavicular notch; harsh, high-pitched, and discontinuous; occur when a patient inhales or exhales
- Bronchial breath sounds—heard above the clavicles on each side of the sternum, between the scapulae, and over the

manubrium; loud, high-pitched, and discontinuous; loudest when the patient exhales

– Bronchovesicular breath sounds — best heard over the upper third of the sternum and between the scapulae; medium pitched and continuous; heard when the patient inhales or exhales

– Vesicular breath sounds — heard over the rest of the lungs; soft and low-pitched; are prolonged during inhalation and shortened during exhalation.

- Classify each sound according to its intensity, location, pitch and duration.
- Note whether the sound occurs when the patient inhales, exhales, or both.
- Diminished but normal breath sounds in both lungs may indicate:
  - emphysema
  - atelectasis
  - severe bronchospasm
  - shallow breathing.
- Breath sounds in only one lung may indicate:
  - pleural effusion
  - pneumothorax
  - tumor
  - mucus plugs.

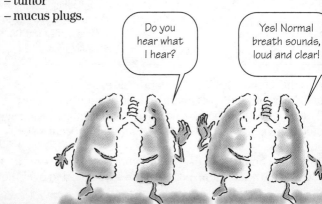

Check the patient for vocal fremitus—voice sounds resulting from chest vibrations that occur as the patient speaks. Abnormal transmission of voice sounds may occur over consolidated areas.

- Bronchophony
- Egophony
- Whispered pectoriloquy

Diagnostic tests, such as arterial blood gas analysis and pulmonary function tests, may be necessary if you note abnormal findings.

Assessing vocal fremitus

Ask the patient to repeat the words below while you listen. Auscultate over an area where you heard abnormally located bronchial breath sounds to check for abnormal voice sounds.

Bronchophony	**Egophony**	**Whispered pectoriloquy**
Ask the patient to say, "ninety-nine." Over normal lung tissue, the words sound muffled. Over consolidated areas, the words sound unusually loud.	• Ask the patient to say, "E." • Over normal lung tissue, the sound is muffled. • Over consolidated lung tissue, it will sound like the letter *a*.	• Ask the patient to whisper, "1, 2, 3." • Over normal lung tissue, the numbers will be almost indistinguishable. • Over consolidated lung tissue, the numbers will be loud and clear.

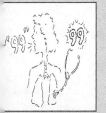
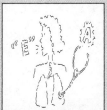
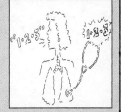

Abnormal findings

Chest-wall abnormalities

- May be congenital or acquired
- May crowd otherwise normal lungs
- May result in a smaller-than-normal lung capacity and limit exercise tolerance
- May increase susceptibility to respiratory failure from a respiratory tract infection

Barrel chest

- Abnormally round and bulging, with a greater-than-normal front-to-back diameter
- May be normal in infants and elderly patients
- Commonly occurs as a result of COPD

Chest deformities

Barrel chest	**Funnel chest**	**Pigeon chest**	**Thoracic kyphoscoliosi**

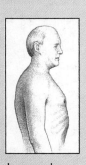 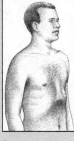 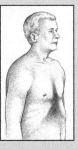 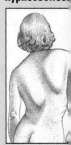

| Increased anteroposterior diameter | Depressed lower sternum | Anteriorly displaced sternum | Raised shoulder and scapula, thoracic convexity, and flared interspaces |

nnel chest

lso known as *pectus excavatum*

efers to a funnel-shaped depression on all or part of the
ternum

Iay interfere with respiratory and cardiac function

May compress the heart and great vessels, causing murmurs

geon chest

lso called *pectus carinatum*

efers to a sternum that protrudes beyond the front of the
bdomen

ncreases the front-to-back diameter of the chest

pracic kyphoscoliosis

)ccurs when the spine curves to one side and the vertebrae
re rotated

Iay be difficult to assess respiratory status because the rota-
on distorts lung tissues

normal respiratory patterns

:hypnea

espiratory rate greater than 20 breaths/minute with shallow
reathing

ommonly seen in patients with:
  restrictive lung disease
  pain
  sepsis
  obesity
  anxiety

Iay be caused by fever (increases by four breaths/minute for
very 1° F [0.6° C] rise in body temperature)

idypnea

espiratory rate below 10 breaths/minute

ypically noted just before a period of apnea or full respirato-
r arrest

Between the lines

Abnormal respiratory patterns

Tachypnea
Shallow breathing with increased respiratory rate

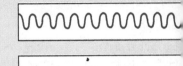

Bradypnea
Decreased rate but regular breathing

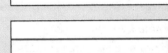

Apnea
Absence of breathing; may be periodic

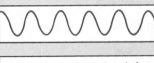

Hyperpnea
Deep, fast breathing

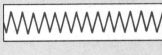

Kussmaul's respirations
Rapid, deep breathing without pauses; breathing usually sounds labored, with deep breaths similar to sighs

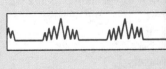

Cheyne-Stokes respirations
Breaths that gradually become faster and deeper than normal and then slower

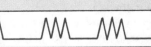

Biot's respirations
Rapid, deep breathing with abrupt pauses between each breath; equal depth to each breath

May occur with central nervous system (CNS) depression as
result of excessive sedation, tissue damage, or diabetic
coma that depresses the brain's respiratory control center

...nea

Absence of breathing
May have short duration
May occur sporadically during:
  Cheyne-Stokes respirations
  Biot's respirations
  other abnormal respiratory patterns
May be life-threatening if periods of apnea last long enough

...perpnea

Deep, rapid breathing
Occurs in patients who exercise or who have anxiety, pain, or
metabolic acidosis
In a comatose patient, may indicate hypoxia or hypoglycemia

...ssmaul's respirations

Rapid, deep, sighing breaths (in adults, more than 20 breaths/
minute)
Occur in patients with metabolic acidosis, especially when associated with diabetic ketoacidosis

...eyne-Stokes respirations

Characterized by a regular pattern of variations in the rate
and depth of breathing; deep breaths alternate with short periods of apnea during a 30- to 170-second period; alternates
with 20- to 60-second periods of apnea
Occur in patients with heart failure, kidney failure, or CNS
damage
May be normal during sleep in children and elderly patients

Biot's respirations

- Rapid, deep breaths that alternate with abrupt periods of apnea
- Ominous sign of severe CNS damage

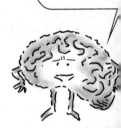

Biot's respirations signal severe CNS damage.

Abnormal breath sounds

- Consider a sound abnormal if it's heard in an area where you would-n't expect to hear it.
- Breath sounds (as well as spoken or whispered words) are louder than normal over areas of consoli-dation because solid tissue trans-mits sound better than air or fluid.
- Breath sounds are muted if the pleural space is filled with pus, fluid, or air.
- If a foreign body or secretions obstruct a bronchus, breath sounds are diminished or absent over lung tissue located di tal to the obstruction.
- Adventitious sounds (crackles, wheezes, rhonchi, stridor, a pleural friction rub) are abnormal anywhere you hear them the lungs.

Crackles

- Brief, intermittent, and nonmusical
- Similar to the sound of static caused by hairs rubbing toget
- Caused by collapsed or fluid-filled alveoli popping open
- Heard primarily when the patient inhales
- Classified as either fine or coarse
  - Fine crackles—typically occur at the lung bases when th patient stops inhaling; occur in restrictive diseases, such as asbestosis, atelectasis, heart failure, pneumonia, pulmonar brosis, and silicosis

- Coarse crackles—may be heard throughout the lungs when the patient starts to inhale and may be present when the patient exhales; occur with bronchiectasis, COPD, or pulmonary edema, and with severely ill patients who can't cough (also referred to as the *death rattle*)
- Usually don't clear with coughing; if they do, they're most likely caused by secretions

Wheezes

- High-pitched, whistling sounds
- Heard first when a patient exhales
- Occur when airflow is blocked
- May also be heard when the patient inhales, if airflow blockage is severe
- Don't change with coughing
- May occur as a result of:
  - asthma
  - infection
  - heart failure
  - airway obstruction from a tumor or foreign body

Signs and symptoms of upper airway obstruction

Anxiety
Dyspnea
Stridor
Wheezing
Decreased or absent breath sounds
Use of accessory muscles
Seesaw movement between chest and abdomen
Inability to speak (complete obstruction)
Cyanosis

Rhonchi
- Low-pitched, snoring, rattling sounds
- Occur primarily when a patient exhales but may also be heard when the patient inhales
- Usually change or disappear with coughing
- Occur when fluid partially blocks the large airways

Stridor
- Loud, high-pitched crowing sound
- Usually heard without a stethoscope during inspiration
- Caused by obstruction in the upper airway
- Requires immediate attention

Pleural friction rub
- Low-pitched, grating, rubbing sound
- Heard when the patient inhales and exhales
- Results from pleural inflammation that causes two layers of pleura to rub together
- Leads to pain in areas where rubbing occurs

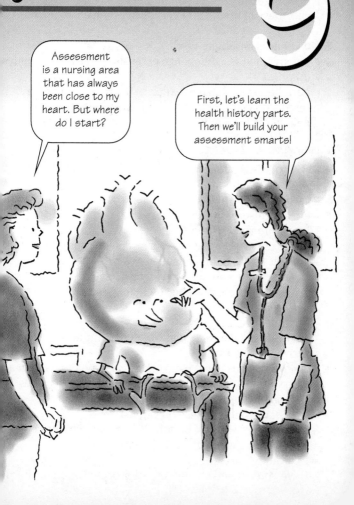

Health history

- Common cardiovascular-related complaints include:
  - chest pain
  - irregular heartbeat or palpitations
  - shortness of breath on exertion or when lying down
  - cyanosis or pallor
  - weakness or fatigue
  - unexplained weight change or swelling of the extremities
  - dizziness
  - peripheral skin changes, such as decreased hair distributi
  altered skin color, or a thin, shiny appearance
  - pain in the extremities, such as leg pain or cramps.

Asking about personal and family health

- Ask for details about family history and past medical histo:
  including a history of:
  - diabetes
  - chronic diseases of the lungs, kidneys, or liver.
- Obtain information about:
  - stress and the patient's mechanisms for coping with it
  - current health habits related to exercise, smoking, and in
  take of alcohol, caffeine, and dietary fat and sodium
  - drugs the patient is taking, including over-the-counter dri
  and herbal preparations
  - previous operations
  - environmental or occupational considerations
  - activities of daily living.
- If the patient has chest pain, ask him to rate the pain on a
  scale of 0 to 10, in which 0 means no pain and 10 means the
  worst pain imaginable.
- Also ask the patient these questions:
  - Are you ever short of breath? If so, what activities cause :
  - Do you ever feel dizzy or fatigued?
  - Do your ankles swell?
  - Have you noticed changes in color or sensation in your le

Physical assessment

Make sure the room is quiet.

Have the patient lie on his back, and position the head of the examination table at a 30- to 45-degree angle.

Assessing the heart

Inspection

Take a moment to assess the patient's general appearance.

Note his skin color, temperature, turgor, and texture.

Note if clubbing is present in the fingers. (Clubbing is a sign of chronic hypoxia caused by a lengthy cardiovascular or respiratory disorder.)

If the patient is dark-skinned, inspect his mucous membranes for pallor.

Inspect the chest.

Note landmarks you can use to describe your findings.

Identifying cardiovascular landmarks

This view of the anterior thorax shows critical landmarks you can use during cardiovascular assessment.

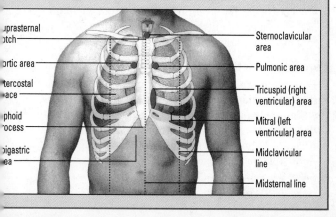

Suprasternal notch

Aortic area

Intercostal space

Xiphoid process

Epigastric area

Sternoclavicular area

Pulmonic area

Tricuspid (right ventricular) area

Mitral (left ventricular) area

Midclavicular line

Midsternal line

– Note structures underlying the chest wall.

– Look for pulsations, symmetry of movement, retractions, heaves (a strong outward thrust of the chest wall that occu during systole).

- Position a light source so that it casts a shadow on the patient's chest.
- Check for the apical impulse.

– The apical impulse should be located at the fifth intercos space at or just medial to the left midclavicular line.

– It can indicate how well the left ventricle is working because the apical impulse corresponds to the apex of the he

– It can be seen in about 50% of adults.

Palpation

- Using the ball of your hand, then your fingertips, gently pa pate over the precordium to find the apical impulse.

– Note heaves or thrills (fine vibrations that feel like the purring of a cat).

– If palpation is difficult with the patient lying on his back, have him lie on his left side or sit upright.

- Palpate the sternoclavicular, aortic, pulmonic, tricuspid, a epigastric areas for abnormal pulsations.

– You normally won't feel pulsations in these areas.

– An aortic arch pulsation in the sternoclavicular area or a abdominal aorta pulsation in the epigastric area may be no mal in a thin patient.

Percussion of the heart

- Percuss at the anterior axillary line and continue toward t sternum along the fifth intercostal space.

– Sound changes from resonance to dullness over the left b der of the heart, normally at the midclavicular line.

– The right border of the heart is usually aligned with the s num and can't be percussed.

scultation for heart sounds

Varm the stethoscope in your hands and then identify the ites where you'll auscultate:
 over the four cardiac valves
 Erb's point (third intercostal space at the left sternal border).
Jse the bell to hear low-pitched sounds and the diaphragm to ear high-pitched sounds.
Auscultate for heart sounds with the patient in three positions:
 lying on his back with the head of the bed raised 30 to 45 degrees
 sitting up
 lying on his left side.
Jse a zigzag pattern over the precordium. You can start at the ase and work downward, or you can start at the apex and work upward.
Listen over the entire precordium, not just over the valves.
Note the heart rate and rhythm.
 Identify S_1 and S_2.
 Listen for adventitious sounds, such as third and fourth eart sounds (S_3 and S_4), murmurs, and rubs.
Auscultate at the aortic area where S_2 is loudest.
 S_2 is best heard at the base of e heart at the end of ventricular systole.
 Sound corresponds to closure f the pulmonic and aortic valves and is generally described as sounding like "dub."
 It's a shorter, higher-pitched, uder sound than S_1.

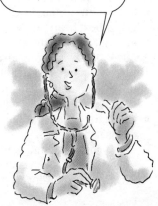

Use the bell of the stethoscope to hear low-pitched heart sounds and the diaphragm to hear high-pitched sounds.

Help desk

Auscultation tips

- Concentrate as you listen for each sound.
- Avoid auscultating through clothing or wound dressings, because these items can block sound.
- Avoid picking up extraneous sounds by keeping the stethoscope tubing off the patient's body and other surfaces.
- Until you become proficient at auscultation, explain to the patient that listening to his chest for a long period doesn't mean that anything is wrong.
- Ask the patient to breathe normally and to hold his breath periodically to enhance sounds that may be difficult to hear.

- When the pulmonic valve closes later than the aortic valv during inspiration, you'll hear a split S_2.
- From the base of the heart, move to the pulmonic area and then down to the tricuspid area.
- Next, move to the mitral area, where S_1 is the loudest.
  - S_1 is best heard at the apex of the heart.
  - Sound corresponds to closure of the mitral and tricuspid valves and is generally described as sounding like "lub."
  - It's low-pitched and dull.
  - S_1 occurs at the beginning of ventricular systole; it may b split if the mitral valve closes just before the tricuspid.
- Listen for S_3 (also called *ventricular gallop* when it occurs adults).
  - S_3 is a normal finding in children and young adults.
  - It's commonly heard in patients with high cardiac output
  - It may be a cardinal sign of heart failure in adults.

ositioning the patient for auscultation

aning forward

an the patient forward to best
ar high-pitched sounds related
 semilunar valve problems, such
 aortic and pulmonic valve mur-
urs. To auscultate for these
unds, place the diaphragm of
e stethoscope over the aortic
d pulmonic areas in the right
d left second intercostal
aces, as shown below.

Left lateral recumbent

The left lateral recumbent position
is best suited for hearing low-
pitched sounds, such as mitral
valve murmurs and extra heart
sounds. To hear these sounds,
place the bell of the stethoscope
over the apical area, as shown
below.

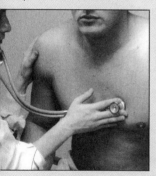
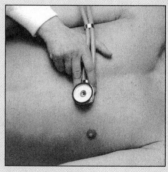

It's best heard at the apex when the patient lies on his left
de.
It's often compared to the y sound in "Ken-tuck-y."
It's low-pitched.
It occurs when the ventricles fill rapidly.
It follows S_2 in early ventricular diastole.
It probably results from vibrations caused by abrupt ventric-
ar distention and resistance to filling.

– It may also be associated with such conditions as pulmonary edema, atrial septal defect, acute myocardial infarction (MI), and the last trimester of pregnancy.
- Listen for S_4 (also called an *atrial gallop*).
   – S_4 is heard over the tricuspid or mitral areas with the patient on his left side.
   – It's heard in patients who are elderly or in those with hypertension, aortic stenosis, or a history of MI.
   – It's commonly described as sounding like "Ten-nes-see."
   – It occurs just before S_1, after atrial contraction.
   – It indicates increased resistance to ventricular filling.
   – It results from vibrations caused by forceful atrial ejection of blood into ventricles that are hypertrophied (enlarged) and don't move or expand as much as they should.

Auscultation for murmurs

- Murmurs occur when:
   – structural defects in the heart chambers or valves cause turbulent blood flow.
   – changes in the viscosity of blood or the speed of blood flow cause turbulence.
- Listen for murmurs over the same precordial areas used in auscultation for heart sounds.
- Murmurs can occur during systole or diastole.
- Murmurs are described using several criteria:
   – pitch (high, medium, or low)
   – intensity (louder or softer)
   – location
   – sound pattern (blowing, harsh, or musical)
   – radiation (to neck or axillae)
   – period during which they occur in the cardiac cycle (pansystolic or midsystolic).
- To better hear murmurs, ask the patient to sit and lean forward or lie on his left side.

Grading murmurs

Use the system outlined here to describe the intensity of a murmur. When recording your findings, use a fraction with roman numerals. The denominator is always VI. For example, a grade III murmur would be recorded as "grade III/VI."

Grade I — barely audible murmur

Grade II — audible but quiet and soft

Grade III — moderately loud, without a thrust or thrill

Grade IV — loud, with a thrill

Grade V — very loud, with a thrust or a thrill

Grade VI — loud enough to be heard before the stethoscope comes to contact with the chest

Auscultation for pericardial friction rub

Have the patient sit upright, lean forward, and exhale.

Listen with the diaphragm of the stethoscope over the third intercostal space on the left side of the chest.

Pericardial friction rub has a scratchy, rubbing quality.

If you suspect a rub but don't hear one, ask the patient to hold his breath.

Assessing the vascular system

Inspection

Start your assessment of the vascular system by making general observations:

Are the arms equal in size?

Are the legs symmetrical?

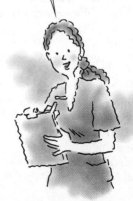

Start your assessment of the vascular system by making general observations.

- Inspect the skin color.
- Note how body hair is distributed.
- Note lesions, scars, clubbing, and edema of the extremities If the patient is confined to bed, check the sacrum for swelling.
- Examine the fingernails and toenails for abnormalities.
- Observe the vessels in the neck.

Carotid artery
- The carotid artery should have a brisk, localized pulsation.
  - Are pulses weak or bounding?
- Carotid pulsation doesn't decrease when the:
  - patient is upright
  - patient inhales
  - carotid is palpated.

Jugular veins
- The internal jugular vein has a softer, undulating pulsation.
- Internal jugular pulsation changes in response to position, breathing, and palpation.
- Inspection of these vessels can provide information about blood volume and pressure in the right side of the heart.
- To check jugular venous pulse, have the patient lie on his back. Elevate the head of the bed 30 to 45 degrees and turn his head slightly away from you.
  - Normally, the highest pulsation occurs no more than 1½″ (4 cm) above the sternal notch; if it appears higher, central nous pressure is elevated and the jugular vein distended.

Palpation
- Assess skin temperature, texture, and turgor.
- Check capillary refill by assessing the nail beds on the fing and toes; refill time should be no more than 3 seconds, or t time that it takes to say "capillary refill."
- Palpate the arms and legs for temperature and edema.
  - Edema is graded on a four-point scale.

- If your finger leaves a slight imprint, the edema is recorded as +1.
- If your finger leaves a deep imprint that only slowly returns to normal, the edema is recorded as +4.

Palpate for arterial pulses by gently pressing with the pads of your index and middle fingers.

- Start at the top of the patient's body at the temporal artery and work your way down.
- Check the carotid, brachial, radial, femoral, popliteal, posterior tibial, and dorsalis pedis pulses.
- Palpate for the pulse on each side, comparing pulse volume and symmetry.
- Don't palpate both carotid arteries at the same time or press too firmly because the patient may faint or become bradycardic.
- Put on gloves when you palpate the femoral arteries.
- All pulses should be regular in rhythm and equal in strength.
- Pulses are graded on a four-point scale: 4+ is bounding, 3+ is increased, 2+ is normal, 1+ is weak, and 0 is absent.

Auscultation

Using the bell of the stethoscope, follow the palpation sequence and listen over each artery.

You shouldn't hear sounds over the carotid arteries.

A hum, or bruit, sounds like buzzing or blowing; it could indicate arteriosclerotic plaque formation.

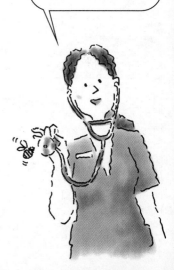

Hear buzzing or blowing upon auscultation? You might have detected a bruit.

Assessing arterial pulses

To assess the arterial pulses, apply pressure with your index and middle fingers.

Carotid pulse
Lightly place your fingers just lateral to the trachea and below the jaw angle. Never palpate both carotid arteries at the same time.

Radial pulse
Apply gentle pressure to the medial and ventral side of the wrist, just below the base of the thumb.

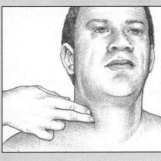

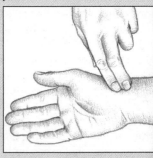

Brachial pulse
Position your fingers medial to the biceps tendon.

Femoral pulse
Press relatively hard at a point inferior to the inguinal ligament.

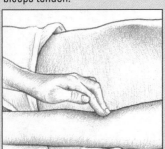

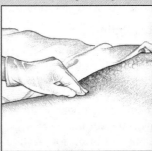

Assessing arterial pulses *(continued)*

Popliteal pulse
Press firmly in the popliteal fossa at the back of the knee.

Dorsalis pedis pulse
Place your fingers on the medial dorsum of the foot.

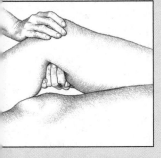

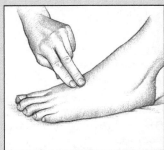

Posterior tibial pulse
Apply pressure behind and slightly below the malleolus of the ankle.

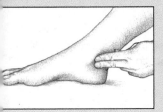

Assess the upper abdomen for abnormal pulsations, which could indicate the presence of an abdominal aortic aneurysm. Auscultate for the femoral and popliteal pulses, checking for a bruit or other abnormal sounds.

Abnormal findings

Chest pain
- Can arise suddenly or gradually
- May be difficult to ascertain a cause initially
- Can radiate to the arms, neck, jaw, or back
- May be steady or intermittent, mild or acute
- Ranges in character from a sharp, shooting sensation to a fe[e]l-
ing of heaviness, fullness, or even indigestion
- May be caused by:
  - angina
  - MI
  - cardiomyopathy
- May be provoked or aggravated by:
  - stress
  - anxiety
  - exertion
  - deep breathing
  - eating certain foods

Fatigue
- Feeling of excessive weariness, lack of energy, or exhausti[on]
accompanied by a strong desire to rest or sleep
- Normal response to:
  - physical overexertion
  - prolonged emotional stress
  - sleep deprivation
- Can be a nonspecific symptom of cardiovascular disease, e[s]-
pecially heart failure and valvular heart disease

Palpitations
- Conscious awareness of one's heartbeat
- Usually felt over the precordium or in the throat or neck
- Described as pounding, jumping, turning, fluttering, or flop-
ping, or as missed or skipped beats

Between the lines

Understanding chest pain

What it feels like	Where it's located	What causes it
Aching, squeezing, pressure, heaviness, and burning pain; usually subsides within 10 minutes	Substernal; may radiate to jaw, neck, arms, and back	Angina pectoris
Tightness or pressure; burning, aching pain, possibly accompanied by shortness of breath, diaphoresis, weakness, anxiety, or nausea; sudden onset; lasts 5 minutes to 2 hours	Typically across chest but may radiate to jaw, neck, arms, or back	Acute MI
Sharp and continuous; may be accompanied by friction rub; sudden onset	Substernal; may radiate to neck or left arm	Pericarditis
Excruciating, tearing pain; may be accompanied by blood pressure difference between right and left arm; sudden onset	Retrosternal, upper abdominal, or epigastric; may radiate to back, neck, or shoulders	Dissecting aortic aneurysm
Sudden, stabbing pain; may be accompanied by cyanosis, dyspnea, or cough with hemoptysis	Over lung area	Pulmonary embolus

(continued)

Understanding chest pain (continued)

What it feels like	Where it's located	What causes
Sudden and severe pain, sometimes accompanied by dyspnea, increased pulse rate, decreased breath sounds (especially on one side), or deviated trachea	Lateral thorax	Pneumothora
Dull, squeezing pain or pressure	Substernal, epigastric areas	Esophageal spasm
Sharp, severe pain	Lower chest or upper abdomen	Hiatal hernia
Burning feeling after eating sometimes accompanied by hematemesis or tarry stools; sudden onset that generally subsides within 15 to 20 minutes	Epigastric	Peptic ulcer
Gripping, sharp pain, possibly accompanied by nausea and vomiting	Right epigastric or abdominal areas; possible radiation to shoulders	Cholecystitis
Continuous or intermittent sharp pain; possibly tender to touch; gradual or sudden onset	Anywhere in chest	Chest-wall syndrome
Dull or stabbing pain usually accompanied by hyperventilation or breathlessness; sudden onset; lasting less than 1 minute or as long as several days	Anywhere in chest	Acute anxie

May be:
- regular or irregular
- fast or slow
- paroxysmal or sustained

May result from:
- cardiac or metabolic disorder
- use of certain drugs
- use of stimulants such as tobacco and caffeine

May occur with a newly implanted prosthetic valve because the valve's clicking sound heightens the patient's awareness of his heartbeat

May be transient, accompanying:
- emotional stress (such as fright, anger, or anxiety)
- physical stress (such as exercise or fever)

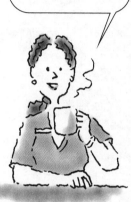

Stimulants such as caffeine and tobacco may lead to palpitations.

Skin and hair abnormalities

Cyanosis, pallor, or cool skin

May indicate poor cardiac output and tissue perfusion

Warmer-than-normal skin

May result from conditions causing fever or increased cardiac output

Absence of body hair on the arms or legs

May indicate diminished arterial blood flow to those areas

Edema (swelling)

May indicate heart failure or venous insufficiency
May result from varicosities or thrombophlebitis

(Text continues on page 164.)

Between the lines

Evaluating cardiovascular findings

Sign or symptom and findings	Probable cause
Fatigue	
• Fatigue following mild activity	Anemia
• Pallor	
• Tachycardia	
• Dyspnea	
• Persistent fatigue unrelated to exertion	Depression
• Headache	
• Anorexia	
• Constipation	
• Sexual dysfunction	
• Loss of concentration	
• Irritability	
• Progressive fatigue	Valvular heart
• Cardiac murmur	disease
• Exertional dyspnea	
• Cough	
• Hemoptysis	
Palpitations	
• Paroxysmal palpitations	Acute anxiety
• Diaphoresis	attack
• Facial flushing	
• Trembling	
• Impending sense of doom	
• Hyperventilation	
• Dizziness	

valuating cardiovascular findings *(continued)*

gn or symptom and findings	Probable cause
alpitations *(continued)*	
Paroxysmal or sustained palpitations	Cardiac arrhythmias
Dizziness	
Weakness	
Fatigue	
Irregular, rapid, or slow pulse rate	
Decreased blood pressure	
Confusion	
Diaphoresis	
Sustained palpitations	Hypoglycemia
Fatigue	
Irritability	
Hunger	
Cold sweats	
Tremors	
Anxiety	
eripheral edema	
Headache	Heart failure
Bilateral leg edema with pitting ankle edema	
Weight gain despite anorexia	
Nausea	
Chest tightness	
Hypotension	
Pallor	
Palpitations	
Inspiratory crackles	

(continued)

Evaluating cardiovascular findings *(continued)*	
Sign or symptom and findings	**Probable cause**
Peripheral edema *(continued)*	
• Bilateral arm edema accompanied by facial and neck edema • Edematous areas marked by dilated veins • Headache • Vertigo • Vision disturbances	Superior vena cava syndrome
• Moderate to severe, unilateral or bilateral leg edema • Darkened skin • Stasis ulcers around the ankle	Venous insufficiency

- Is generalized and accompanied by ascites with chronic right-sided heart failure
- Occurs in lower legs with right-sided heart failure

Abnormal pulsations

Displaced apical impulse
- May indicate an enlarged left ventricle, which may be caused by heart failure or hypertension

Forceful apical impulse
- Lasts longer than one-third of the cardiac cycle
- May point to increased cardiac output

Pulsation in the aortic, pulmonic, or tricuspid area
- May indicate heart chamber enlargement or valvular disease
- If in aortic area only, may also indicate increased cardiac output or an aortic aneurysm

indings in arterial and venous insufficiency

ssessment findings differ in patients with arterial insufficiency and ose with chronic venous insufficiency. These illustrations show those fferences.

rterial insufficiency
- Pulses may be decreased or bsent.
- Skin will be cool, pale, and hiny.
- Pain may be present in the legs nd feet.
- Ulcerations typically occur in e area around the toes, and the ot usually turns deep red when ependent.
- Nails may be thick and ridged.

Chronic venous insufficiency
- Ulcerations occur around the ankle.
- Pulses are present but may be difficult to find because of edema.
- The foot may become cyanotic when dependent.

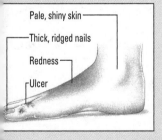

Pale, shiny skin
Thick, ridged nails
Redness
Ulcer

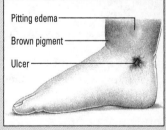

Pitting edema
Brown pigment
Ulcer

igastric pulsation

May indicate early heart failure or an aortic aneurysm

lsation in the sternoclavicular area

uggests an aortic aneurysm

ght pulsations in the right and left sternum

May occur with anemia, anxiety, increased cardiac output, or thin chest wall

Weak arterial pulse
- May indicate decreased cardiac output or increased peripheral vascular resistance
- Points to arterial atherosclerotic disease

Strong or bounding pulsations
- Usually occur in patients with conditions that causes increased cardiac output, such as hypertension, hypoxia, anemia, exercise, or anxiety

Thrill
- A palpable vibration
- Usually suggests a valvular dysfunction

Heave
- Lifting of the chest wall felt during palpation
- If along the left sternal border, may mean right ventricular hypertrophy
- If over the left ventricular area, may mean a ventricular aneurysm

Abnormal sounds

Murmurs

Low-pitched murmur
- Occurs with aortic stenosis, a condition in which the aortic valve calcifies and restricts blood flow
- Characterized as harsh and midsystolic
- Radiates from the valve to the carotid artery
- Shifts from crescendo (increasing intensity) to decrescend (decreasing intensity) and back

Between the lines

Recognizing abnormal heart sounds

When auscultation reveals an abnormal heart sound, try to identify the sound and its timing in the cardiac cycle. Knowing those characteristics can help you identify the possible cause of the sound.

Abnormal heart sound	Timing	Possible causes
Accentuated S_1	Beginning of systole	Mitral stenosis or fever
Diminished S_1	Beginning of systole	Mitral insufficiency, heart block, or severe mitral insufficiency with a calcified, immobile valve
Split S_1	Beginning of systole	Right bundle-branch block (BBB) or premature ventricular contractions
Accentuated S_2	End of systole	Pulmonary or systemic hypertension
Diminished or inaudible S_2	End of systole	Aortic or pulmonic stenosis
Persistent S_2 split	End of systole	Delayed closure of the pulmonic valve, usually from overfilling of the right ventricle, which causes prolonged systolic ejection time

Recognizing abnormal heart sounds *(continued)*

Abnormal heart sound	Timing	Possible causes
Reversed or paradoxical S_2 split that appears during exhalation and disappears during inspiration	End of systole	Delayed ventricular stimulation, left BBB, or prolonged left ventricular ejection time
S_3 (ventricular gallop)	Early diastole	Overdistention of ventricle during the rapid-filling segment of diastole or mitral insufficiency of ventricular failure (normal in children and young adults)
S_4 (atrial or presystolic gallop)	Late diastole	Pulmonic stenosis, hypertension, coronary artery disease, aortic stenosis, or forceful atrial contraction because of resistance to ventricular filling late in diastole (resulting from left ventricular hypertrophy)
Pericardial friction rub (grating or leathery sound at the left sternal border; usually muffled, high-pitched, and transient)	Throughout systole and diastole	Pericardial inflammation

- Results from the turbulent, high-pressure flow of blood across stiffened valves and through a narrowed opening

dium-pitched murmur

Occurs with pulmonic stenosis, a condition that develops
when the pulmonic valve calcifies and interferes with blood
flow out of the right ventricle
Occurs near the pulmonic valve
Characterized as harsh and systolic
Shifts from crescendo to decrescendo and back
Caused by turbulent blood flow across a stiffened, narrowed
valve

h-pitched murmur

Occurs with:
  aortic insufficiency, a condition in which the blood flows
backward through the aortic valve
  pulmonic insufficiency, a condition in which the blood flows
backward through the pulmonic valve
Characterized as blowing, decrescendo, and diastolic
With aortic insufficiency, radiates from the aortic valve area
to the left sternal border
With pulmonic insufficiency:
  Can be heard at Erb's point (at the left sternal border of the
third intercostal space)
  Is high-pitched only if the patient has a higher-than-normal
pulmonary pressure

nbling murmur

Occurs with mitral stenosis, a condition in which the mitral
valve calcifies and blocks blood flow out of the left atrium
Characterized as low-pitched, rumbling, and crescendo-
decrescendo in the mitral valve area
Results from turbulent blood flow across the stiffened, narrowed valve

wing murmur

Occurs with mitral insufficiency, a condition in which blood
regurgitates into the left atrium

– Characterized as high-pitched and blowing throughout systole (pansystolic or holosystolic)
– May radiate from the mitral area to the left axillary line
– Heard best at the apex

Low, rumbling murmur

- Occurs with tricuspid stenosis, a condition in which the tricuspid valve calcifies and blocks blood flow through the valve from the right atrium
- Characterized as crescendo-decrescendo in the tricuspid area
- Results from turbulent blood flow across the stiffened, narrowed valvular leaflets

High-pitched, blowing murmur

- Occurs with tricuspid insufficiency, a condition in which blood regurgitates into the right atrium
- Occurs throughout systole in the tricuspid area
- Becomes louder when the patient inhales

Bruits

- Murmurlike sound of vascular (rather than cardiac) origin
- If heard during arterial auscultation, murmurs may indicate
  – occlusive arterial disease
  – arteriovenous fistula
- Caused by various high cardiac output conditions such as anemia, hyperthyroidism, and pheochromocytoma

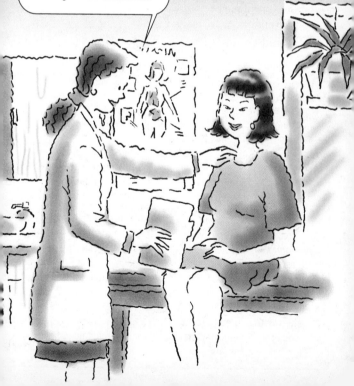

Health history

Asking about the chief complaint

- Common complaints about the breasts include:
  - pain
  - nipple discharge
  - rash
  - lumps
  - masses
  - other changes.
- Ask about the sign or symptom's onset, duration, and sever
  - Ask women what day of the menstrual cycle the signs or symptoms appear?
  - What relieves or worsens them?

Male concerns

Breasts in boys

- Estrogen, which is produced in males *and* females, may temporarily stimulate breast tissue in adolescent boys.
- Breast enlargement usually stops when boys begin producing adequate amounts of the male sex hormone testosterone.

Gynecomastia

- Older men may have gynecomastia (abnormal breast enlargement).
- Possible causes include:
  - age-related hormonal alterations or a hormonal imbalance
  - certain medications

- cirrhosis
- leukemia
- thyrotoxicosis
- hormone administration
- illicit drug use (especially ma ijuana and heroin)
- alcohol consumption.

Male breast cancer

- Breast cancer in men usually occurs in the areolar area.
- Examine a man's breasts thoroughly during a complete physic assessment.
  - Palpate the nipple and areol
  - Assess for the same change you would in a woman.

sking about medical history

Ask the patient whether she has ever had breast lumps, biopsy, or surgery, including enlargement or reduction.
- If she has had breast cancer, fibroadenoma, or fibrocystic disease, ask for more information.

Ask about her menstrual cycle.
- Record the date of her last menses.

Ask about pregnancies.
- How many pregnancies?
- How many live births?
- How old was she each time she became pregnant?
- Did she have complications?
- Did she breast-feed?

Ask if any family members have had breast disorders, especially breast cancer.
- Having a close relative with breast cancer greatly increases the patient's risk of having the disease.

Ask the patient about the incidence of other types of cancer in her family.

Teach the patient how to examine her breasts and about the importance of regular breast examinations and mammograms.

sking about current health

Ask the patient how old she is (some breast changes are age-related).

Ask her to describe breast changes in detail, if she noticed any.
- When did they occur?
- Does she have pain, tenderness, discharge, or rash?
- Has she had changes in her underarm area?

Ask the patient what drugs she takes regularly. (Birth control medications can cause breast swelling and tenderness.)

Ask about diet, especially caffeine intake. (Caffeine has been linked to fibrocystic disease of the breasts.)

Ask the patient if she's under a lot of stress, smokes, or drinks alcohol. (Links exist between those factors and breast cancer.)

Physical assessment

- Provide privacy.
- Make the patient as comfortable as possible.
- Explain what the examination involves.

Examining the breasts

- Make sure the room is well lit.
- Have the patient disrobe from the waist up and sit with her arms at her sides.
- Keep both breasts uncovered so you can observe them simultaneously to detect differences.

Inspection

- Skin should be:
  - smooth
  - undimpled
  - the same color as the rest of the skin.
- Check for edema, which can accompany lymphatic obstruction and may signal cancer.
- Note breast size and symmetry.
  - Asymmetry may occur normally in some adult women, with the left breast usually larger than the right.
- Inspect the nipples.
  - Note size and shape.
  - If inverted (dimpled or creased), ask the patient when she first noticed the inversion.
- To detect skin or nipple dimpling that might not have been obvious before, inspect the breasts while the patient:
  - holds her arms over her head
  - has her hands on her hips.

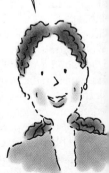

Dimples may be a good feature for smile, but they shouldn't appear on the breasts.

f the patient has large or pendulous breasts, have her stand
with her hands on the back of a chair and lean forward.
— This position helps reveal subtle breast or nipple asymmetry.

lpation

Ask the patient to lie in a supine position.
Place a small pillow under her shoulder on the side you're examining; doing so causes the breast on that side to protrude.
Have the patient put her hand behind her head on the side
you're examining.
— This position spreads the breast more evenly across the
chest and makes finding nodules easier).
f the breasts are small, the patient can leave her arm at her
side.
Perform palpation.

---

alpating the breast

Use your three middle fingers to
palpate the breast systematically.
Rotate your fingers gently
against the chest wall, moving in
concentric circles.
Include the tail of Spence in
your examination.

Examining the areola and nipple

• Palpate the areola and nipple.
• Gently squeeze the nipple
between your thumb and index
finger to check for discharge.

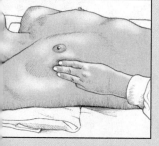
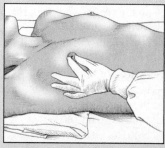

– Place your fingers flat on the breast and compress the tissues gently against the chest wall.

– Palpate in concentric circles outward from the nipple.

– Palpate the entire breast, including the periphery, tail of Spence, and areola.

– If the breasts are pendulous, palpate down or across the breast with the patient sitting upright.

- Note the consistency of the breast tissue—normal consistency varies widely, depending in part on the proportions of fat and glandular tissue.

- Check for nodules and unusual tenderness—tenderness may be related to cysts and cancer.

- Ask the patient where she is in her menstrual cycle; nodularity, fullness, and mild tenderness are also premenstrual symptoms.

- A lump or mass that feels different from the rest of the breast tissue may indicate a pathologic change and warrants further investigation by a doctor.

- If you find what you think is an abnormality, check the other breast, too.

- The inframammary ridge at the lower edge of the breast is normally firm and may be mistaken for a tumor.

- If you palpate a mass, record these characteristics:

  – size in centimeters

  – shape (round, discoid, regular, or irregular)

  – consistency (soft, firm, or hard)

  – mobility

  – degree of tenderness

  – location, using the quadrant or clock method.

- Palpate the nipple.

  – Note its elasticity; it should be rough, elastic, and round.

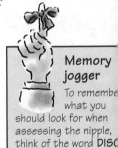

Memory jogger

To remember what you should look for when assessing the nipple, think of the word DISC

Discharge

Inversion

Skin changes

Contrast with the other side.

Identifying locations of breast lesions

Mentally divide the breast into four quadrants and a fifth segment, the tail of Spence.

Describe your findings according to the appropriate quadrant or segment.

You can also think of the breast as a clock, with the nipple in the center. Then specify locations according to the time (2 o'clock, for example).

Specify the location of a lesion or other findings by the distance in centimeters from the nipple.

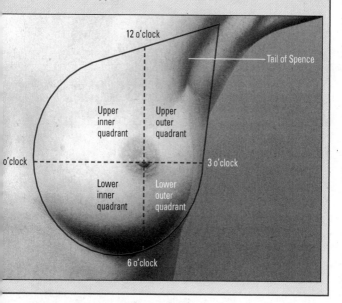

It should protrude from the breast.

Compress the nipple and areola to detect discharge.

If discharge is present and the patient isn't pregnant or lactating, assess the color, consistency, and quantity of discharge and obtain a cytologic smear.

– Put on gloves.
– Place a glass slide over the nipple.
– Smear the discharge on the slide.
– Spray the slide with a fixative.
– Label the slide with the patient's name and the date.
– Send the slide to the laboratory, according to facility polic

Examining the axillae

- With the patient sitting or standing, inspect the skin of the a
  illae for rashes, infections, or unusual pigmentation.
- To perform palpation:
  – Ask the patient to relax her arm on the side you're examin
  ing before palpating.
  – Support her elbow with one of your hands.
  – Cup the fingers of your other hand, and reach high into th
  apex of the axilla.
  – Place your fingers directly behind the pectoral muscles,
  pointing toward the midclavicle.

Palpating the axillae

- Have the patient sit or lie down.
- Wear gloves if an ulceration or discharge is present.
- Ask the patient to relax her arm, and support it with your nondominant hand.
- Keep the fingers of your dominant hand together.
- Reach high into the apex of the axilla, as shown at right.
- Position your fingers so they're

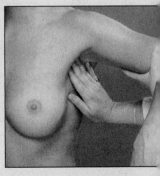

directly behind the pectoral muscles, pointing toward the midclavicle
- Sweep your fingers downward against the ribs and serratus anterie muscle to palpate the midaxillary or central lymph nodes.

sessing the axillary nodes

'alpate the central nodes by pressing your fingers downward
nd in toward the chest wall.

ou can usually palpate one or more of the nodes, which
hould be soft, small, and nontender.

ry to palpate the other groups of lymph nodes for compari-
on if you feel a hard, large, or tender lesion.

alpate the pectoral and anterior nodes.

Grasp the anterior axillary fold between your thumb and
ngers.

Palpate inside the borders of the pectoral muscles.

alpate the lateral nodes.

Press your fingers along the upper inner arm.

Compress these nodes against the humerus.

alpate the subscapular or posterior
odes.

Stand behind the patient.

Press your fingers to feel the inside of
e muscle of the posterior axillary fold.

sessing the clavicular nodes

ssess these nodes if the axillary nodes
ppear abnormal.

 assess clavicular nodes:

Have the patient relax her
eck muscles by flexing her
ead slightly forward.

Stand in front of her and hook
our fingers over the clavicle
side the sternocleidomastoid
uscle.

Rotate your fingers deeply
to this area to feel the supra-
avicular nodes.

> If the axillary nodes appear abnormal, palpate the clavicular nodes.

Abnormal findings

- The menstrual cycle, certain prescription drugs, pregnancy and other conditions can cause breast changes.

Breast nodule

- Lump that may be found in any part of the breast, including the axilla
- May be benign lump of fibrocystic breast disease or malign mass of breast cancer

Dimpling

- Puckering or retraction of skin on the breast
- Results from abnormal attachment of the skin to underlyin tissue
- Suggests an inflammatory or malignant mass beneath the s surface
- Usually represents a late sign of breast cancer

Peau d'orange

- Late sign of breast cancer
- Involves edematous thickening and pitting of breast skin
- Can also occur with breast or axillary lymph node infection of Graves' disease
- Resembles an orange peel
- Stems from lymphatic edema around deepened hair follicles

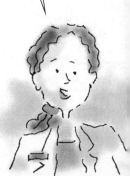

Peau d'orange isn't an "a-peeling" finding. It's a late sig of breast cancer.

Nipple retraction

- Inward displacement of the nipple below the level of surrounding breast tissue

Dimpling and peau d'orange

Dimpling

Dimpling usually suggests an inflammatory or malignant mass beneath the skin's surface. The illustration below shows breast dimpling and nipple inversion caused by a malignant mass above the areola.

Peau d'orange

• Peau d'orange (shown below) is usually a late sign of breast cancer.
• It can also occur with breast or axillary lymph node infection.
• The orange-peel appearance comes from lymphatic edema around deepened hair follicles.

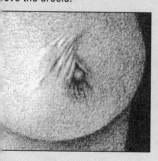

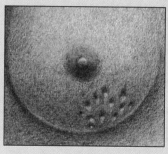

• may indicate an inflammatory breast lesion or cancer
• results from scar tissue formation within a lesion or large mammary duct, which pulls tissue inward, causing nipple deviation, flattening, and finally retraction

Nipple discharge

• can occur spontaneously or can be elicited by nipple stimulation
• characterized as intermittent or constant, as unilateral or bilateral, and by color, consistency, and composition
• may be a normal finding
• can signal serious underlying disease, particularly when accompanied by other breast changes
• typically caused by:

Between the lines

Evaluating breast findings

Sign or symptom and findings	Probable cau‹

Breast dimpling
- Firm, irregular, nontender lump   Breast absce‹
- Nipple retraction, deviation, inversion, or flattening
- Enlarged axillary lymph nodes

- History of trauma to fatty tissue of the breast   Fat necrosis
(patient may not remember such trauma)
- Tenderness and erythema
- Bruising
- Hard, indurated, poorly delineated lump that's fibrot-
ic and fixed to underlying tissue or overlying skin
- Nipple retraction

- Heat   Mastitis
- Erythema
- Swelling
- Pain and tenderness
- Flulike signs and symptoms, such as fever, malaise,
fatigue, and aching

Breast nodule
- Single nodule that feels firm, elastic, and   Adenofibrom‹
round or lobular, with well-defined margins
- Extremely mobile, "slippery" feel
- No pain or tenderness
- Size varies from that of a pinhead to very large
- Grows rapidly
- Usually located around the nipple or the lateral side
of the upper outer quadrant

valuating breast findings *(continued)*

gn or symptom and findings	Probable cause
reast nodule *(continued)* Hard, poorly delineated nodule Fixed to the skin or underlying tissue Breast dimpling Nipple deviation or retraction Almost one-half are located in the upper outer adrant Nontender Serous or blood discharge Edema or peau d'orange of the skin overlying the ass Axillary lymphadenopathy	Breast cancer
Smooth, round, slightly elastic nodules Increase in size and tenderness just before men-ruation Mobile Clear, watery (serous), or sticky nipple discharge Bloating Irritability Abdominal cramping	Fibrocystic breast disease
reast pain Tender, palpable abscesses on the periphery the areola Fever Inflamed sebaceous Montgomery's glands	Areolar gland abscess

(continued)

endocrine disorders
cancer
certain drugs
blocked lactiferous ducts

Evaluating breast findings *(continued)*

Sign or symptom and findings	Probable cau
Breast pain *(continued)*	
• Unilateral breast pain or tenderness • Serous or bloody nipple discharge, usually only from one duct • Small, soft, poorly delineated mass in the ducts beneath the areola	Intraductal papilloma
• Small, well-delineated nodule • Localized erythema • Induration	Sebaceous cyst (infectio
Nipple retraction	
• Unilateral nipple retraction • Hard, fixed, nontender breast nodule • Nipple itching, burning, or erosion • Watery or bloody nipple discharge • Altered breast contour • Dimpling or peau d'orange • Tenderness, redness, and warmth	Breast cance
• Unilateral nipple retraction, deviation, cracking, or flattening • Firm and indurated or tender, discrete breast nodule • Warmth, erythema, tenderness, and edema • Possible fatigue, fever, and chills	Mastitis

Breast pain

- Commonly results from benign breast disease, such as mastis or fibrocystic breast disease
- May occur during rest or movement
- May be aggravated by manipulation or palpation
- Classified as tenderness if pain is elicited by physical conta

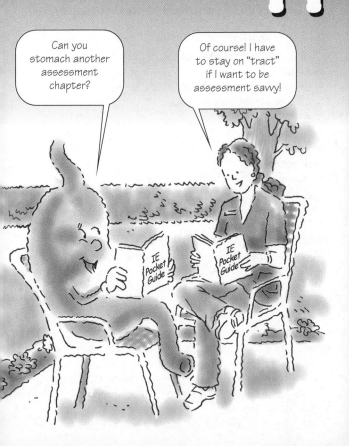

Health history

- Common GI complaints include:
  - pain
  - heartburn
  - nausea and vomiting
  - altered bowel habits.
- Ask the patient about the location, quality, onset, duration, frequency, and severity of each of his symptoms.

Asking about past health

- Ask about past GI illnesses, such as:
  - ulcer
  - liver, pancreas, or gallbladder disease
  - inflammatory bowel disease
  - rectal or GI bleeding
  - hiatal hernia
  - irritable bowel syndrome
  - diverticulitis
  - gastroesophageal reflux disease
  - cancer.
- Ask about abdominal surgery or trauma.

Asking about current health

- Ask the patient if he's taking any medications.
  - Several drugs — especially nonsteroidal anti-inflammatory drugs, aspirin, antibiotics, and opioid analgesics — can cause nausea, vomiting, and other GI signs and symptoms.
  - Habitual laxative use may cause constipation.
- Ask about allergies to medications or foods.
- Ask about changes in appetite, difficulty chewing or swallowing, and changes in bowel habits.
  - Does the patient have excessive belching or passing of gas?
  - Has he noticed a change in the color, amount, and appearance of his stools?
  - Has he ever seen blood in his stools?

f the patient's chief complaint is diarrhea, find out if he recently traveled abroad.

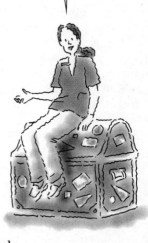

Traveling abroad can affect GI health if a patient is exposed to contaminated food or water.

sking about family health

Ask the patient whether anyone in his family has had a GI disorder.
Ask about disorders with a familial link, such as:
- ulcerative colitis
- colorectal or gastric cancer
- peptic ulcers
- diabetes
- alcoholism
- Crohn's disease.

sking about psychosocial ealth

Inquire about other factors that may affect GI health, such as:
- home life
- food and exercise habits
- oral hygiene
- occupation and financial situation
- recent life changes and stress level
- alcohol, caffeine, and tobacco use.

Different strokes

Culture and GI tract history

Patients from Japan, Iceland, Chile, and Austria are at higher risk for death from gastric cancer than patients from other countries.
Crohn's disease is more common in patients who are Jewish.

Physical assessment

- Assessment should include a thorough examination of the mouth, abdomen, and rectum.
- Explain the techniques you'll be using and let the patient know that some procedures might be uncomfortable.
- Perform the examination in a private, quiet, warm, and well lit room.

Examining the mouth

- Use inspection and palpation.
- Put on gloves before examining the patient.
- Inspect the mouth and jaw for asymmetry and swelling.
- Check the patient's bite.
  - Note malocclusion from an overbite or underbite.
- Inspect the inner and outer lips, teeth, gums, and oral muco with a penlight.
  - Note bleeding; ulcerations; carious, loose, missing, or broken teeth; and color changes, including rashes.
- Palpate the gums, inner lips, and cheeks for tenderness, lumps, and lesions.
- Assess the tongue.
  - Check for coating, tremors, swelling, and ulcerations.
  - Note unusual breath odors.
- Examine the pharynx.
  - Press a tongue blade firmly down on the middle of the tongue and ask the patient to say "Ahh."
  - Look for uvular deviation, tonsillar abnormalities, lesions, plaques, and exudate.

Examining the abdomen

- Use this sequence for examination: inspection, auscultation percussion, and palpation (palpating or percussing the abdomen before you auscultate can change the character of th patient's bowel sounds and lead to an inaccurate assessmen

Abdominal quadrants

To perform a systematic GI assessment, visualize the abdominal structures in four quadrants, as shown here.

Right upper quadrant
- Right lobe of liver
- Gallbladder
- Pylorus
- Duodenum
- Head of pancreas
- Hepatic flexure of colon
- Portions of ascending and transverse colons

Left upper quadrant
- Left lobe of liver
- Stomach
- Body of pancreas
- Splenic flexure of colon
- Portions of transverse and descending colons

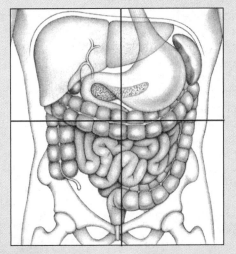

Right lower quadrant
- Cecum and appendix
- Portion of ascending colon

Left lower quadrant
- Sigmoid colon
- Portion of descending colon

- Take these actions before the examination:
  – Ask the patient to empty his bladder.
  – Drape the genitalia and, if the patient is female, her breast
  – Place a small pillow under the patient's knees to help rela
  the abdominal muscles.
  – Ask the patient to keep his arms at his sides.
  – Keep the room warm. Chilling can cause abdominal musc
  to become tense.
  – Warm your hands and the stethoscope.
  – Ask the patient to point to any painful areas. Assess those
  areas last to help prevent the patient from becoming tense.

Inspection

- Mentally divide the abdomen into four quadrants and then
  imagine the organs in each quadrant.
- Know these three terms to help you pinpoint your physical
  findings:
  – epigastric (above the umbilicus and between costal margins)
  – umbilical (around the navel)
  – suprapubic (above the symphysis pubis).
- Observe the abdomen for symmetry.
- Check for bumps, bulges, or masses. (A bulge
  may indicate bladder distention or hernia.)
- Observe abdominal shape and contour.
  – The abdomen should be flat to
  rounded in people of average weight
  and may be slightly concave in a
  slender person.
  – It may protrude with obesity, pregnancy, ascites (a large accumulation
  of fluid in the peritoneal cavity), or
  abdominal distention.
- Assess the umbilicus.

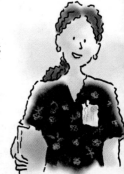

Remember
to assess
painful area
last.

It should be inverted and located midline in the abdomen.

It may protrude with pregnancy, ascites, an underlying mass, or an umbilical hernia (assess while the patient raises his head and shoulders).

Skin should be smooth and uniform in color.

Striae, or stretch marks, can be caused by pregnancy, excessive weight gain, or ascites.

New striae are pink or blue.

Old striae are silvery white.

In patients with dark skin, striae may be dark brown.

Note dilated veins.

Record the length of any surgical scars on the abdomen.

Note abdominal movements and pulsations.

Usually, waves of peristalsis can't be seen; if they're visible, they look like slight, wavelike motions.

Visible rippling waves may indicate bowel obstruction and should be reported immediately.

In thin patients, pulsation of the aorta is visible in the epigastric area.

Marked pulsations may occur with hypertension, aortic insufficiency, aortic aneurysm, and other conditions causing widening pulse pressure.

Auscultation

Lightly place the stethoscope diaphragm in the right lower quadrant, slightly below and to the right of the umbilicus.

Auscultate in a clockwise fashion in each of the four quadrants.

Note the character and quality of bowel sounds in each quadrant.

You may need to auscultate for 5 minutes before you hear sounds.

Allow enough time to listen in each quadrant before you decide that bowel sounds are absent.

Briefly clamp the tube or turn off suction before auscultating the abdomen of a patient with a nasogastric tube or anoth-

Listening for vascular sounds

Use the bell of your stethoscope to auscultate for vascular sounds at the sites shown in the illustration.

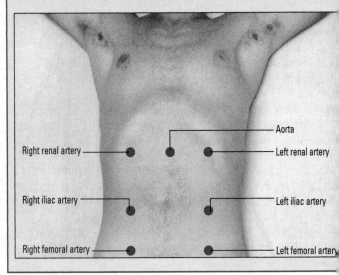

Aorta

Right renal artery — — Left renal artery

Right iliac artery — — Left iliac artery

Right femoral artery — — Left femoral artery

er abdominal tube (suction noises can obscure or mimic ac
al bowel sounds).
- Normal bowel sounds are high-pitched, gurgling noises caused by air mixing with fluid during peristalsis.
- Borborygmus, or stomach growling, is the loud, gurgling, splashing bowel sound heard over the large intestine as gas passes through it.
- Bowel sounds are classified as normal, hypoactive, or hyperactive.
  – Hyperactive bowel sounds — loud, high-pitched, tinkling sounds that occur frequently — may be caused by diarrhea, constipation, or laxative use.

- Hypoactive bowel sounds are heard infrequently and indicate diminished peristalsis; they're associated with ileus, bowel obstruction, peritonitis, torsion of the bowel, or the use of opioid analgesics and other medications.

Using firm pressure, listen with the bell of the stethoscope over the aorta and renal, iliac, and femoral arteries for bruits, venous hums, and friction rubs.

Percussion

Direct or indirect percussion is used to detect:
- the size and location of abdominal organs
- air or fluid in the abdomen, stomach, or bowel.

To perform direct percussion, strike your hand or finger directly against the patient's abdomen.

To perform indirect percussion, use the middle finger of your dominant hand or a percussion hammer to strike a finger resting on the patient's abdomen.

Begin percussion in the right lower quadrant and proceed clockwise, covering all four quadrants.

Percussing the abdomen

Don't percuss the abdomen of a patient with an abdominal aortic aneurysm or a transplanted abdominal organ; doing so can precipitate a rupture or organ rejection.

Two sounds are normally heard:
- Tympany is a clear, hollow sound like a drum beating, which is heard over hollow organs, such as an empty stomach or bowel.
- Dullness (muffled sound) is heard over solid organs, such as the liver, kidney, or feces-filled intestines.

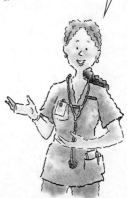

Percussion can be used to detect air or fluid in the abdomen, stomach, or bowel.

Percussing the liver
- Percussion of the liver can help you estimate its size.

Percussing the spleen
- The spleen is located at about the level of the 10th rib, at the left midaxillary line.
- It usually can't be percussed because tympany from the colon masks the dullness of the spleen.
- Percussion may produce a small area of dullness, generally (17.8 cm) or less in adults.
- To check for splenomegaly:
  - Ask the patient to breathe deeply.
  - Percuss along the 9th to 11th intercostal spaces on the left
  - Listen for a change from tympany to dullness—a sign of splenic enlargement.

Percussing and measuring the liver

- Start in the right midclavicular line in an area of lung resonance, and percuss downward toward the liver.
- Identify the upper border of the liver when you hear dullness (muffled sounds).
- Use a pen to mark the spot where the sound changes to dullness.
- Start in the right midclavicular line at a level below the umbilicus, and lightly percuss upward toward the liver.

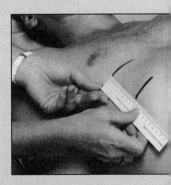

- Mark the spot where the sound changes from tympany to dullness.
- Use a ruler to measure the vertical span between the two marked spots, as shown.
- In an adult, a normal liver span ranges from 2½″ to 4¾″ (6.5 to 12 cm).

- Measure the area of dullness.

Palpation

Abdominal palpation includes light and deep touch that helps:
- determine the size, shape, position, and tenderness of major abdominal organs
- detect masses and fluid accumulation.

Palpate all four quadrants, leaving painful and tender areas for last.

Light palpation helps identify:
- muscle resistance and tenderness
- location of some superficial organs.

Palpate using standard techniques.
- Put the fingers of one hand close together.
- Depress the skin about ½" (1.5 cm) with your fingertips.

Palpating the liver

- Place the patient in the supine position.
- Standing at his right side, place your left hand under his back at the approximate location of the liver.
- Place your right hand slightly below the liver's upper border (indicated by the line in the illustration at right).
- Point the fingers of your right hand toward the patient's head just under the right costal margin.

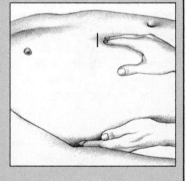

- As the patient inhales deeply, gently press in and up on the abdomen until you feel the liver under your right hand; the edge should be smooth, firm, and somewhat round.
- Note any tenderness.

– Make gentle, rotating movements.
– Avoid short, quick jabs.
- The abdomen should be soft and nontender.
- Note organs, masses, and areas of tenderness or resistance
  – Determine whether resistance is because the patient is co
  tense, or ticklish, or if it's because of involuntary guarding c
  rigidity from muscle spasms or peritoneal inflammation.
  – Help the ticklish patient relax by putting his hand over yo
  as you palpate.
  – If the patient complains of abdominal tenderness before y
  touch him, palpate by lightly placing your stethoscope on h
  abdomen.
- To perform deep palpation:
  – Push down the abdomen 2″ to 3″ (5 to 7.5 cm).
  – If the patient is obese, put one hand on top of the other
  and push.
  – Palpate the entire abdomen in a clockwise
  direction, checking for tenderness, pulsations, organ enlargement, and masses.
- If the patient's abdomen is rigid, don't
  palpate it. Peritoneal inflammation may be
  present. Palpation could cause pain or could
  rupture an inflamed organ.
- Palpate the patient's liver to
  check for enlargement and
  tenderness.
- Keep in mind that you can't
  detect the spleen by palpation
  unless it's enlarged. If you feel
  it, stop palpating immediately
  because compression can
  cause rupture.

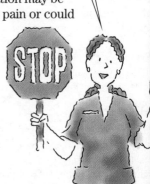

Don't palpate a rigi abdomen.

ecial assessment procedures

erform the test for rebound tenderness when you suspect eritoneal inflammation.
- Do this test at the end of your examination.
- Choose a site away from the painful area.
- Position your hand at a 90-degree angle to the abdomen.
- Push down slowly and deeply into the abdomen.
- Withdraw your hand quickly; rapid withdrawal causes the nderlying structures to rebound suddenly and results in a harp, stabbing pain on the inflamed side.
- Don't repeat this maneuver because you may rupture an in- amed appendix.

scites can be caused by advanced liver disease, heart fail- re, pancreatitis, or cancer.
- To assess ascites, measure the fullest part of the abdomen vith a tape measure.
- Mark the assessment point on the patient's abdomen with ndelible ink.
- Consistent measurement is important, especially if paracen- esis, or fluid removal, is performed.

hecking for ascites

Have an assistant place the nar edge of her hand firmly on e patient's abdomen at its mid- e.

As you stand facing the patient's ead, place the palm of your ght hand against the patient's ft flank.

Give the right abdomen a firm p with your left hand, as own.

If ascites is present, you may e and feel fluid rippling across the abdomen.

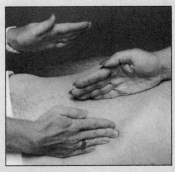

Examining the rectum and anus

- Perform a rectal examination if the patient is age 40 or olde
- Explain the procedure to the patient.
- Inspect the perianal area.
- Put on gloves and spread the buttocks to expose the anus a surrounding tissue.
- Check for fissures, lesions, scars, inflammation, discharge, rectal prolapse, and external hemorrhoids.
- Ask the patient to strain as if he's having a bowel movemen this may reveal internal hemorrhoids, polyps, or fissures.
- Skin in the perianal area is normally somewhat darker than that of the surrounding area.
- Apply a water-soluble lubricant to your gloved index finger.
- Tell the patient to relax and let him know that he'll feel som pressure.
- Ask the patient to bear down.
- As the sphincter opens, gently insert your finger into the re tum, toward the umbilicus.
- Rotate your finger clockwise and then counterclockwise to palpate as much of the rectal wall as possible (the rectal wa should feel soft and smooth, without masses, fecal impacti or tenderness).
- Remove your finger from the rectum.
- Inspect the glove for stools, blood, and mucus.
- Test fecal matter adhering to the glove for occult blood usir a guaiac test.

Abnormal findings

Nausea and vomiting

Usually occur together
May be caused by:
- acute pancreatitis
- appendicitis
- intestinal obstruction
- cholecystitis (inflammation of the gallbladder)
- gastric and peritoneal irritation
- myocardial infarction
- neurologic disturbances
- some medications

Dysphagia

Difficulty swallowing
May be accompanied by weight loss
May be caused by:
- achalasia of the lower esoph-
agogastric junction
- neurologic disease, such as
stroke or Parkinson's disease
- obstruction
Can lead to aspiration and
pneumonia

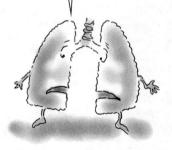

Patients with dysphagia are at risk for aspiration and pneumonia? That fact is hard for me to swallow!

Skin color changes

Cullen's sign

Refers to a bluish umbilicus
Indicates intra-abdominal hemorrhage

Turner's sign

Bruising on the flank
Indicates retroperitoneal hemorrhage

Between the lines

Evaluating GI findings

Sign or symptom and findings	Probable cause
Diarrhea	
• Soft, unformed stools or watery diarrhea that may be foul-smelling or grossly bloody • Abdominal pain, cramping, and tenderness • Fever	*Clostridium difficile* infection
• Diarrhea that occurs within several hours of ingesting milk or milk products • Abdominal pain, cramping, and bloating • Borborygmi • Flatus	Lactose intolerance
• Recurrent bloody diarrhea with pus or mucus • Hyperactive bowel sounds • Occasional nausea and vomiting	Ulcerative colitis
Rectal bleeding	
• Moderate to severe rectal bleeding • Epistaxis • Purpura	Coagulation disorders
• Bright-red rectal bleeding with or without pain • Diarrhea or ribbon-shaped stools • Possible grossly bloody stools • Weakness and fatigue • Abdominal aching and dull cramps	Colon cancer
• Chronic bleeding with defecation • Painful defecation	Hemorrhoids

Evaluating GI findings *(continued)*

Sign or symptom and findings	Probable cause
Nausea and vomiting	
Nausea and vomiting that follow or accompany abdominal pain Pain that progresses rapidly to severe, stabbing pain in the right lower quadrant (McBurney's sign) Abdominal rigidity and tenderness Constipation or diarrhea Tachycardia	Appendicitis
Nausea and vomiting of undigested food Diarrhea Abdominal cramping Hyperactive bowel sounds Fever	Gastroenteritis
Nausea and vomiting Headache with severe, constant, throbbing pain Fatigue Photophobia Light flashes Increased noise sensitivity	Migraine headache

Abdominal redness
May indicate inflammation

Dilated, tortuous, visible abdominal veins
May indicate inferior vena cava obstruction

Cutaneous angiomas
May signal liver disease

Constipation

- Can be caused by:
  - immobility
  - sedentary lifestyle
  - medications
- May be accompanied by complaints of:
  - dull ache in the abdomen
  - full feeling
  - hyperactive bowel sounds, which may be caused by irritable bowel syndrome
- Can occur with complete intestinal obstruction (patient can't pass flatus or stools and doesn't have bowel sounds below the obstruction)
- Occurs more commonly in older patients

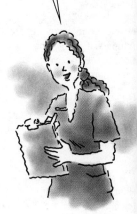

Constipation may be accompanied by a dull ache in the abdomen and a full feeling.

Diarrhea

- May be caused by:
  - GI conditions such as Crohn's disease
  - medications
  - toxins (when patient has a fever)
- May be accompanied by:
  - abdominal tenderness
  - anorexia
  - cramping
  - hyperactive bowel sounds

Distention

- May occur with:
  - colon filled with feces
  - gas
  - tumor

May be caused by an incisional hernia, which may protrude when the patient lifts his head and shoulders

Abnormal bowel sounds

Hyperactive

Indicate increased intestinal motility
Have many causes, including laxative use, gastroenteritis, and life-threatening intestinal obstruction

Hypoactive

Can be caused by full colon, paralytic ileus, and recent bowel surgery

Between the lines

Interpreting abnormal bowel sounds

Sound and description	Possible cause
Abnormal bowel sounds in any quadrant	
Hyperactive sounds (unrelated to hunger)	Diarrhea, laxative use, or early intestinal obstruction
Hypoactive, then absent sounds	Paralytic ileus or peritonitis
High-pitched tinkling sounds	Intestinal fluid and air under tension in a dilated bowel
High-pitched rushing sounds coinciding with abdominal cramps	Intestinal obstruction

Splenomegaly

- Spleen enlargement
- May be caused by:
  - mononucleosis
  - trauma
  - illnesses that destroy red blood cells, such as sickle cell anemia and some cancers

Hepatomegaly

- Liver enlargement
- May be caused by:
  - hepatitis
  - cirrhosis
  - poorly controlled diabetes
  - amyloidosis
  - hepatic abscess
  - leukemia
  - lymphoma
  - obesity

Friction rubs

- Can occur over the liver and spleen in the epigastric region
- May indicate splenic infarction or hepatic tumor

Abdominal bruits

- May be caused by aortic aneurysms or partial arterial obstruction

Abdominal pain

- May be caused by:
  - appendicitis
  - cholecystitis
  - intestinal obstruction
  - other inflammatory disorders
  - peritonitis
  - ulcers

Between the lines

Assessing abdominal pain

If your patient complains of abdominal pain, ask him to describe the pain. Ask him how and when it started. This table will help you assess the pain and determine possible causes.

Type of pain	Possible cause
Burning	Peptic ulcer or gastroesophageal reflux disease
Cramping	Biliary colic, irritable bowel syndrome, diarrhea, constipation, or flatulence
Severe cramping	Appendicitis, Crohn's disease, or diverticulitis
Stabbing	Pancreatitis or cholecystitis

If abdominal pain occurs 1½ to 3 hours after eating, it indicates a duodenal ulcer.

• May occur with rebound tenderness, which can be caused by peritonitis or appendicitis
• When caused by a duodenal ulcer:
– presents as gnawing pain in the midepigastrium
– occurs 1½ to 3 hours after the patient has eaten
– may awaken the patient
– may be relieved by antacids or food

Hematochezia

- Passage of bloody stools
- Usually indicates — and may be the first sign of — GI bleeding
- May also result from:
  - anal fissure
  - colitis
  - colorectal cancer
  - Crohn's disease
  - hemorrhoids

Female genitourinary system

12

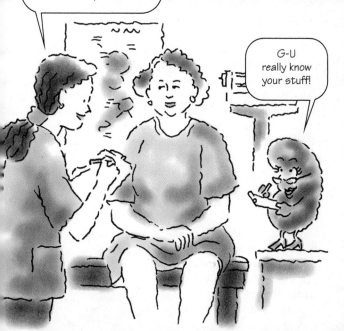

Health history

- Because the urinary and reproductive systems are located so close to each other, you and your patient may have trouble differentiating whether signs and symptoms originate in the urinary tract or reproductive system.
- Investigate minor complaints.
- Ask about the problem's onset, duration, and severity.
- Ask about measures taken to treat the problem.

Asking about the urinary system

- The most common urinary system complaints include:
  – output changes, such as polyuria, oliguria, and anuria
  – voiding pattern changes, such as hesitancy, frequency, urgency, nocturia, and incontinence
  – changes in urine color
  – pain.
- Ask about past illnesses and preexisting conditions that can affect a patient's urinary tract health.
  – Has the patient ever had a urinary tract infection (UTI)?
  – Has the patient ever had renal calculi or kidney trauma? (Either can alter the structure and function of the kidneys and bladder.)
- Make a list of all the prescribed medications, herbal preparations, and over-the-counter drugs the patient takes.
  – Some drugs can affect the appearance of urine.
  – Nephrotoxic drugs can alter urinary function.
- Ask about current problems.
  – Does she have diabetes, cardiovascular disease, or hypertension?

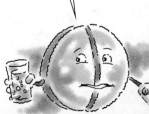

Find out if the patient is taking nephrotoxic drugs. These drugs can alter urinary function.

Has she noticed a change in the color or odor of her urine?
Does she have pain or burning during urination?
Does she have problems with incontinence or frequency?
Does she have allergies?
Ask about family history to obtain information about her risk of developing kidney failure or kidney disease.

Asking about the reproductive system

The most common reproductive system complaints are:
- pain
- vaginal discharge
- abnormal uterine bleeding
- pruritus
- infertility.

Focus on the patient's current complaints, and then explore her reproductive, sexual-social, and family history.

Ask her to describe symptoms in her own words, encouraging her to speak freely.

Start with less-personal questions to establish rapport.

Ask about her menstrual cycle.
How old was she when she began to menstruate?
How long does menstruation usually last? (Normal duration is 2 to 8 days.)
How often does it occur? (Normal cycle for menstruation is one menses every 21 to 38 days.)
Does she have cramps, spotting, or an unusually heavy or light flow?

Different strokes

Cultural differences in menstruation

Black girls tend to have longer menses and heavier menstrual blood flow than White girls of the same age.

- Spotting between menses, or metrorrhagia, may be normal patients taking low-dose hormonal contraceptives or proge terone; otherwise, spotting may indicate infection, cancer, other abnormality.
- Menses generally starts by age 15; if it hasn't and if no secondary sex characteristics have developed, the patient sho be evaluated by a doctor.
- When the patient seems comfortable, ask her about her sex al practices, including:
  - number of sexual partners she currently has
  - whether she experiences pain with intercourse
  - if she has ever had an STD
  - her human immunodeficiency virus status.
- Ask her when her last Papanicolaou (Pap) test was. What the result?
- Ask the patient if she has ever been pregnant.
  - How many times has she been pregnant and how many times did she give birth?
  - Has she had any miscarriages or therapeutic abortions?
  - Did she have a vaginal or cesarean delivery for each birth
  - What kind of birth control, if any, does she use?
- If she's sexually active, talk to her about the importance of safer sex and the prevention of STDs.
- If postmenopausal, ask for the date of her last menses.
- To find out about menopausal symptoms, ask her if she's having:
  - hot flashes
  - night sweats
  - mood swings
  - flushing
  - vaginal dryness or itching.
- Ask if she has questions or concerns.

Physical assessment

Examining the urinary system

Your patient's vital signs, weight, and mental status provide clues about renal dysfunction.

Inspection

Observe the color and shape of the area around the kidneys and bladder.
Skin should be free from:
- lesions
- discolorations
- inflammation
- swelling.

Palpation

Kidneys

Kidneys usually aren't palpable unless they're enlarged.
You may be able to palpate both kidneys in elderly patients because of decreased muscle tone and elasticity.
Enlarged kidneys may indicate:
- hydronephrosis
- cysts
- tumors.

Bladder

The bladder can be palpated only if it's distended.
To palpate the bladder:
- Ask the patient to lie in a supine position.
- Use the fingers of one hand to palpate the lower abdomen in a light dipping motion.
- A distended bladder:
- feels firm and relatively smooth
- extends above the symphysis pubis.

Palpating the kidneys

- Have the patient lie in a supine position.
- Stand next to her right side to palpate the right kidney.
- Place your left hand under her back and your right hand on her abdomen.
- Instruct the patient to inhale deeply, so her kidney moves downward.
- Press up with your left hand and down with your right as the patient inhales, as shown.

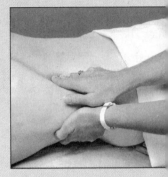

- Reach across the patient's abdomen, placing your left hand behind her left flank to palpate the left kidney.
- Place your right hand over the area of the left kidney.
- Ask the patient to inhale deeply again.
- Pull up with your left and press down with your right as she inhales.

- If the patient is 12 or more weeks pregnant, you may feel th fundus of the uterus, palpable just above the symphysis pu bis.

Percussion

Kidneys
- Percuss the kidneys to check for costovertebral angle tend ness that occurs with inflammation.
  - Have the patient sit up.
  - Place the ball of your nondominant hand on her back at t costovertebral angle of the 12th rib.
  - Strike the ball of that hand with the ulnar surface of your dominant hand.
  - Use just enough force to cause a painless but perceptible thud.

Bladder

Ask the patient to empty her bladder.

Have her lie in the supine position.

Start at the symphysis pubis and percuss upward toward the bladder and over it.

You should hear tympany; dull sound signals retained urine.

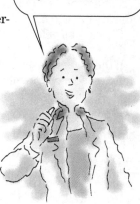

Percussing a dull sound over the bladder signals retained urine.

Examining the reproductive system

Ask the patient to void to prevent discomfort and inaccurate findings during palpation.

Have her disrobe and put on an examination gown.

Explain the procedure to the patient before the examination.

Help her into the dorsal lithotomy position.

Drape all areas not being examined.

Examine the external genitalia. (The internal genitalia are examined only by advanced practice nurses.)

Inspecting the external genitalia

Put on a pair of gloves.

Spread the labia and locate the urethral meatus.

The urethral meatus should be a pink, irregular, slitlike opening at the midline, just above the vagina.

Note the presence of discharge (a sign of urethral infection) or ulcerations (signs of an STD).

Inspect the external genitalia and pubic hair to assess sexual maturity.

Using your index finger and thumb, gently spread the labia majora and minora.

The area should be moist and free from lesions.

– You may detect a normal discharge that varies from clear and stretchy before ovulation to white and opaque after ovu tion; it should be odorless and nonirritating to the mucosa.

- Examine the vestibule, especially the area around the Bartholin's and Skene's glands.
  – Check for swelling, redness, lesions, discharge, and unusu odor.
  – If these abnormal conditions exist, notify the doctor and c tain a specimen for culture.
- Inspect the vaginal opening, noting whether the hymen is ii tact or perforated.

Palpating the external genitalia

- Spread the labia with one hand and palpate with the other.
  – Labia should feel soft and the patient shouldn't feel any pain.
  – Note swelling, hardness, or tenderness.
  – If you detect a mass or lesion, palpate it to determine the size, shape, and consistency.
- If you find swelling or tenderness, see if you can palpate Bartholin's glands, which normally aren't palpable.
  – Insert your finger carefully into the patient's posterior int tus, and place your thumb along the lateral edge of the swollen or tender labium.
  – Gently squeeze the labium.
  – If discharge from the duct results, culture it.
- If the urethra is inflamed, milk it and the area of Skene's glands.
  – Moisten your gloved index finger with water.
  – Separate the labia with your other hand, and insert your i dex finger about $1\frac{1}{4}''$ (3 cm) into the anterior vagina.
  – With the pad of your finger, gently press and pull outwaro
  – Continue palpating down to the introitus; this procedure shouldn't cause the patient discomfort.
  – Culture the discharge.

Abnormal findings

Many patients with urinary disorders don't realize they're ill because they have only mild signs and symptoms or no symptoms at all.

Disorders of the genitourinary system can have wide-ranging effects on other body systems.

Ovarian dysfunction can alter hormonal balance.

Kidney dysfunction can alter blood pressure, disrupt serum electrolytes, and affect production of red blood cells.

Urinary abnormalities

Polyuria

Production and excretion of more than 2,500 ml of urine daily

Fairly common finding

Usually results from:
- diabetes insipidus
- diabetes mellitus
- diuretic use

May be caused by:
- psychological, neurologic, or renal disorders
- urologic disorders, such as pyelonephritis and postobstructive uropathy
- increases risk of developing hypovolemia

Hematuria

Presence of blood in the urine

Causes brown or bright-red urine

Timing suggests the location of the underlying problem

At the start of urination, indicates a disorder of the urethra

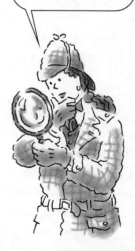

Determining at what point during urination hematuria occurs can provide clues to the underlying problem.

– At the end of urination, signifies a disorder of the bladder neck

– Throughout urination, indicates a disorder located above the bladder neck

• Can also be caused by GI, vaginal, or certain coagulation disorders

Urinary frequency

• Abnormally frequent urination
• Commonly results from decreased bladder capacity
• Is a classic symptom of a UTI
• Also occurs with urethral stricture, neurologic disorders, pregnancy, and uterine tumors

Urinary urgency

• Sudden urge to urinate
• Accompanied by bladder pain in many cases
• Is another common symptom of a UTI
• Can be painful even with small amounts of urine in the bladder because inflammation decreases bladder capacity
• May occur without pain, possibly indicating an upper motor neuron lesion that affects bladder control

Urinary hesitancy

• Difficulty starting a urine stream
• Can occur with:
  – UTI
  – partial obstruction of the lower urinary tract
  – neuromuscular disorders
  – use of certain drugs

Nocturia

• Excessive urination at night
• Common sign of kidney or lower urinary tract disorders

Can result from:
- disruption of the normal urine patterns
- overstimulation of the nerves and muscles that control urination
- cardiovascular, endocrine, or metabolic disorders
- use of diuretics

Urinary incontinence

- Common complaint
- May be transient or permanent
- Involves the release of small or large amounts of urine
- May be caused by:
- stress incontinence
- tumor
- bladder cancer
- calculi
- neurologic disorders, such as Guillain-Barré syndrome, multiple sclerosis, and spinal cord injury

Dysuria

- Pain during urination
- Signals a lower UTI
- Onset of pain suggests the cause
- If just before urination, indicates bladder irritation or distention
- If at the start of urination, usually signals a bladder outlet obstruction
- If at the end of urination, can be a sign of bladder spasm
- If throughout urination, may indicate pyelonephrosis, especially when fever, chills, hematuria, and flank pain are also present

(Text continues on page 221.)

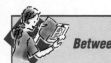

Between the lines

Evaluating female genitourinary findings

Sign or symptom and findings	Probable caus
Dysmenorrhea	Endometriosis
• Steady, aching pain that begins before menses and peaks at the height of menstrual flow; may occur between menses	
• Pain may radiate to the perineum or rectum	
• Premenstrual spotting	
• Dyspareunia	
• Infertility	
• Nausea and vomiting	
• Tender, fixed adnexal mass palpable on bimanual examination	
• Severe abdominal pain	Pelvic inflammatory disease
• Fever	
• Malaise	
• Foul-smelling, purulent vaginal discharge	
• Menorrhagia	
• Cervical motion tenderness and bilateral adnexal tenderness on pelvic examination	
• Cramping pain that begins with menstrual flow and diminishes with decreasing flow	Premenstrual syndrome
• Abdominal bloating	
• Breast tenderness	
• Depression	
• Irritability	
• Headache	
• Diarrhea	

Evaluating female genitourinary findings *(continued)*

Sign or symptom and findings	Probable cause
Dysuria	
Urinary frequency	Cystitis
Nocturia	
Straining to void	
Hematuria	
Perineal or lower back pain	
Fatigue	
Low-grade fever	
Dysuria throughout voiding	Urinary system
Bladder distention	obstruction
Diminished urine stream	
Urinary frequency and urgency	
Sensation of bloating or fullness in the lower abdomen or groin	
Urinary urgency	UTI
Hematuria	
Bladder spasms	
Feeling of warmth or burning during urination	
Urinary incontinence	
Urge or overflow incontinence	Bladder cancer
Hematuria	
Dysuria	
Nocturia	
Urinary frequency	
Suprapubic pain from bladder spasms	
Palpable mass on bimanual examination	

(continued)

Evaluating female genitourinary findings *(continued)*

Sign or symptom and findings	Probable caus
Urinary incontinence *(continued)* • Overflow incontinence • Painless bladder distention • Episodic diarrhea or constipation • Orthostatic hypotension • Syncope • Dysphagia	Diabetic neuropathy
• Urinary urgency and frequency • Sensory impairment • Constipation • Muscle weakness • Emotional lability	Multiple sclerosis
Vaginal discharge • Profuse, white, curdlike discharge with a yeasty, sweet odor • Exudate may be lightly attached to the labia and vaginal walls • Vulvar redness and edema • Intense labial itching and burning • External dysuria	Candidiasis
• Yellow, mucopurulent, odorless, or acrid discharge • Dysuria • Dyspareunia • Vaginal bleeding after douching or coitus	*Chlamydia* infection
• Yellow or green, foul-smelling discharge that can be expressed from the Bartholin's or Skene's ducts • Dysuria • Urinary frequency and incontinence • Vaginal redness and swelling	Gonorrhea

enital abnormalities

enital lesions

Syphilitic chancre
- Causes a red, painless, eroding lesion with a raised, indurated border (in the early stages)
- Usually appears inside the vagina but may also appear on the external genitalia

Genital warts
- Are an STD caused by human papillomavirus
- Produce painless warts on the vulva, vagina, cervix, or anus
- Start as tiny red or pink swellings that grow and develop stemlike structures
- Commonly result in multiple swellings with a cauliflower appearance

Genital herpes
- Produces multiple shallow vesicles, lesions, or crusts inside the vagina, on the external genitalia, on the buttocks and, sometimes, on the thighs
- May cause dysuria, regional lymph node inflammation, pain, edema, and fever
- Appears on Pap test as multinucleated giant cells with intranuclear inclusion bodies

Vaginitis usually results from overgrowth of infectious organisms.

ginitis

Usually results from overgrowth of infectious organisms
Causes redness, itching, dyspareunia (painful intercourse), dysuria, and a malodorous discharge

- Bacterial vaginosis
  - Causes a fishy odor
  - Produces a thin, grayish white discharge
- *Candida albicans*
  - A fungal infection
  - Causes pruritus and a thick, white, curdlike discharge that appears in patches on the cervix and vaginal walls
  - Has a yeastlike odor
- Trichomoniasis
  - May cause an abundant malodorous discharge that's either yellow or green and frothy or watery
  - Involves redness and possibly red papules on the cervix and vaginal walls, giving the tissue a "strawberry" appearance
- *Chlamydia trachomatis*
  - Causes a mucopurulent cervical discharge and cystitis
  - Produces no symptoms in 75% of infected women
- Gonorrhea
  - Commonly produces no symptoms
  - May cause a purulent green-yellow discharge and cystitis.

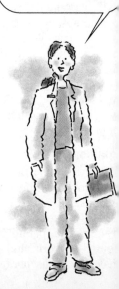

Chlamydia trachomatis produces no symptoms in 75% of infected women.

Cervical lesions

- Translucent nodules located on the cervical surface, known as *retention cysts*, have no pathologic significance
- If hard, granular, and friable during speculum examination, may indicate late-stage cervical cancer

Cervical polyps

Bright red, soft, and fragile
Usually benign
May bleed
Usually rise from the endocervical canal

Cervical cyanosis

May accompany any disorder that causes systemic hypoxia or venous congestion in the cervix
Common during pregnancy
May be observed in women using hormonal contraceptives

Vaginal prolapse

Also called *cystocele*
Occurs when the anterior vaginal wall and bladder prolapse into the vagina
Appears as pouch or bulging on the anterior wall as the patient bears down during speculum examination

Uterine prolapse

Occurs when uterus prolapses into the vagina
May even be visible outside the body

Rectocele

Herniation of the rectum through the posterior vaginal wall
Appears as a pouch or bulging on the posterior wall as the patient bears down

Menstrual abnormalities

Dysmenorrhea

Painful menstruation
Affects more than 50% of menstruating women
Usually characterized by mild to severe cramping or colicky pain in the pelvis or lower abdomen that may radiate to the thighs and lower sacrum
Gradually subsides as bleeding tapers off

Amenorrhea

- Absence of menstrual flow
- Can be classified as primary or secondary
  - Primary amenorrhea—menstruation fails to begin before age 16
  - Secondary amenorrhea—menstruation begins at an appropriate age but later ceases for 3 or more months in the absence of normal physiologic causes, such as pregnancy, lactation, or menopause
- May result from:
  - anovulation
  - physical obstruction to menstrual outflow, such as from an imperforate hymen, cervical stenosis, or intrauterine adhesions
  - drug or hormonal treatments

Male genitourinary system

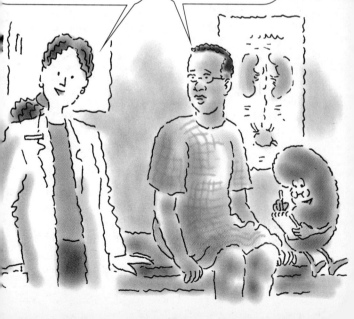

13

Health history

- As you obtain a patient's health history, remember that he may feel uncomfortable discussing genitourinary (GU) problems and having intimate areas of his body examined. These tips may help:
  - Be aware of your own feelings about sexuality.
  - If you appear comfortable discussing the patient's problem, he'll be encouraged to talk openly.
- Common patient complaints related to the urinary system include:
  - pain during urination
  - changes in voiding pattern
  - changes in urine color
  - changes in urine output.
- Common complaints related to the reproductive system include:
  - penile discharge
  - erectile dysfunction
  - infertility
  - scrotal or inguinal masses
  - pain
  - tenderness.

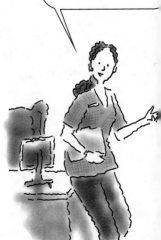

If you appear comfortable, your patient may feel more at ease when discussing GU problems.

Asking about past health and family health

- Ask the patient about his medical history, especially about presence of diabetes or hypertension.
- Also ask the following questions:
  - Did you ever have kidney or bladder trauma or kidney stones?
  - Have you ever had a kidney or bladder infection or an infection of the reproductive system?

Help desk

Putting your patient at ease

Make sure that the room is private and that you won't be interrupted.
Tell the patient that his answers will remain confidential, and phrase your questions tactfully.
Start with less sensitive topics and then move to more sensitive topics such as sexual function.
Don't rush or omit important facts because the patient seems embarrassed.
Be especially tactful with older men.
– They may see a normal decrease in sexual prowess as a sign of declining health.
– They may be less willing to talk about sexual problems than younger men are.
When asking questions, keep in mind that many men view sexual problems as a sign of diminished masculinity.
– Phrase your questions carefully.
– Offer reassurance as needed.
Consider the patient's educational and cultural background.
– If he uses slang or euphemisms to talk about his sexual organs or function, confirm that you're both talking about the same thing.

– Have you had any medical condition that required catheterization?

Inquire about his family's health to learn about any increased risk of developing renal failure or kidney disease.

Asking about current health

Ask the patient about his current GU health status.
Begin by asking if he has been circumcised. If not, ask if he can retract and replace the prepuce (foreskin) easily.
– Inability to retract the prepuce is called *phimosis*.

Assessing urine appearance

While taking the patient's health history, ask him if he has noticed any change in the color of his urine. Use this chart to help interpret any changes.

Change	Possible causes
Pale and diluted	Diabetes insipidus, diuretic therapy, or excessive fluid intake
Concentrated and dark yellow or amber	Acute febrile disease, inadequate fluid intake, or severe diarrhea or vomiting
Blue-green	Methylene blue ingestion
Green-brown	Bile duct obstruction
Dark brown or black	Acute glomerulonephritis or intake of drugs such as chlorpromazine
Orange-red or orange-brown	Obstructive jaundice, urobilinuria, intake of drugs such as rifampin or phenazopyridine
Red or red-brown	Hemorrhage, porphyria, or intake of drugs such as phenazopyridine

  – Inability to replace the prepuce is called *paraphimosis*.
  – If left untreated, phimosis and paraphimosis can impair local circulation and lead to edema and gangrene.
- Inquire whether the patient has noticed sores, lumps, or ulcers on his penis. These signs can indicate a sexually transmitted disease (STD).
- Ask the patient if he has scrotal swelling. This condition may indicate:
  – hematocele

- testicular tumor
- epididymitis
- inguinal hernia.

Ask whether he has penile discharge or bleeding.

Ask what medications the patient regularly takes. Be sure to ask about:
- over-the-counter drugs
- prescription drugs
- herbal preparations
- illicit drugs.

king about sexual health and practices

Ask about his sexual preference and practices so that you can assess risk-taking behaviors.

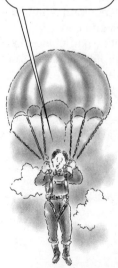

Assess the patient's risk-taking behaviors and talk to him about preventing risks.

- How many sexual partners does he have now?
- How many has he had in the past?
- Has he ever had an STD? If so, did e receive treatment for it?
- What precautions, if any, does he take to prevent contracting STDs?
- What's his human immunodeficiency virus status?
- Does he use birth control measures? If so, what kind?
- Has he had a vasectomy?

Ask the patient about his sexual health.
- Has he ever had trauma to his penis or scrotum?
- Was he ever diagnosed with an undescended testicle?
- Has he ever been diagnosed with low sperm count? If so, explain that hot baths, frequent bicycle or

Help desk

Teaching about testicular self-examination

- Have the patient hold his penis out of the way with one hand.
- Instruct him to roll each testicle between the thumb and first two fingers of his other hand.
  - A normal testicle should have no lumps, move freely in the scrotal sac, and feel firm, smooth, and rubbery.
  - Both testicles should be the same size, although the left one is usually lower than the right because the left spermatic cord is longer.
- If abnormalities are found, the patient should notify his doctor immediately.

motorcycle riding, and tight underwear or athletic supporters can elevate scrotal temperature and temporarily decrease sperm count.

- If he participates in sports, ask how he protects himself from potential genital injuries.
- Ask whether he knows how to examine his testicles for signs of testicular cancer.
  - The patient should perform self-examination monthly.
  - Testicular cancer, the most common type of cancer in men ages 20 to 35, can be treated successfully when it's detected early.

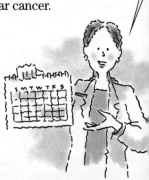

Instruct your male patients to perform monthly testicular self-examinations.

hysical assessment

xamining the urinary system

Before examining specific structures, check the patient's
blood pressure and weight.

Observe the patient's skin.

- Decreased renal function may cause pale skin because of a
low hemoglobin level or even uremic frost (snowlike crystals
on the skin created by metabolic wastes).

Look for signs of fluid imbalance, including:

- dry mucous membranes
- sunken eyeballs
- edema
- ascites.

Before performing an assessment:

- ask the patient to urinate
- help him lie down in the supine position with his arms at his
sides.

Expose only the areas being examined.

spection

Inspect the abdomen, which should be symmetrical and
smooth, flat, or concave (when supine).

Inspect the patient's skin. His skin should be free from lesions, bruises, discolorations, and prominent veins.

Watch for abdominal distention with tight, glistening skin and
striae (silvery streaks caused by rapidly developing skin ten-
sion). These signs indicate ascites, which may accompany
nephrotic syndrome.

rcussion and palpation

Tell the patient what you're going to do during the examination. Otherwise, he may be startled and you could mistake his
reaction for a feeling of acute tenderness.

Performing fist percussion

- Ask the patient to sit up with his back to you.
- Explain that you'll be gently striking his back.
- Place one hand at the costovertebral angle and strike it with the ulnar surface of your other hand, as shown at right.

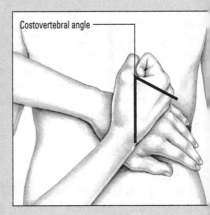

Costovertebral angle

- Percuss the kidneys. Ask about and note any patient reactio that indicates he might feel pain or tenderness; these signs could suggest a kidney infection.
- Percuss the bladder to assess for tympany or dullness. A dul sound, instead of the normal tympany, may indicate retainec urine in the bladder caused by bladder dysfunction or infection.
- Palpate the bladder to check for distention.
- Check the size of the kidneys. Enlargement may accompany hydronephrosis, a cyst, or a tumor. Keep in mind that the ki neys aren't usually palpable.

Auscultation

- Auscultate the renal arteries to rule out bruits, which signal renal artery stenosis.

amining the reproductive system

ut on gloves.

lake the patient as comfortable as possible.

xplain what you're doing before performing each step.

lake sure that the privacy curtain is fully drawn or that the
oor is closed to help the patient feel less self-conscious.

pection

is

nspect the penis.
- Size depends on the patient's age and
verall development.
- Skin should be slightly wrinkled.
- Skin color should be pink to light
rown in white patients and light
rown to dark brown in black pa-
ents.

heck the penile shaft for le-
ions, nodules, inflammation,
nd swelling.

spect the glans for dis-
harge, genital warts, inflam-
ation, lesions, swelling, and
megma (a cheesy secretion
ommonly found beneath the
repuce).

Inspect the glans of an un-
ircumcised penis by retract-
g the prepuce.

pen the urethral meatus by
ently compressing the tip of
e glans.

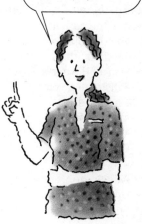

To inspect the
glans of an
uncircumcised penis,
you need to retract
the prepuce.

- It should be located in the center of the glans.
- It should be pink and smooth.

btain a culture specimen if you note discharge.

Examining the urethral meatus

To inspect the urethral meatus, compress the tip of the glans, as shown.

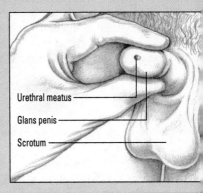

Urethral meatus

Glans penis

Scrotum

Scrotum and testicles
- Ask the patient to hold his penis away from his scrotum so you can observe the scrotum's general size and appearance
  - Skin on the scrotum is darker than on the rest of the body.
- Spread the surface of the scrotum and examine the skin for
  - distended veins
  - nodules
  - redness
  - sebaceous cysts (firm, white to yellow, cutaneous lesions that aren't tender are a normal finding)
  - swelling
  - ulceration.
- Check for pitting edema, a sign of cardiovascular disease.
- Spread the pubic hair and check the skin for lesions and parasites.
- If the patient is a child, check especially for penile enlargement.

ssessing pediatric patients

ps and techniques

Before palpating a boy's scro-
m during a testicular examina-
on, explain what you'll be doing
nd why.
Keep in mind that a younger
hild may want his parent present
r comfort; whereas an older boy
ill probably want privacy.
Make sure the patient is com-
rtably warm and as relaxed as
ssible.
– Cold and anxiety may cause
his testicles to retract. When
this happens, you can't palpate
them.

Hernia and hydroceles

• If you see an enlarged scrotum
in a boy younger than age 2, suspect a scrotal extension of an
inguinal hernia, a hydrocele, or
both.
 – Hydroceles, usually associated with inguinal hernias, are
 common in children of this age-
 group.
 – A hydrocele isn't tender or
 reducible, and you can transilluminate it.

Obesity

• An adolescent boy who's obese
may appear to have an abnormally
small penis.
• You may need to retract the fat
pad over the symphysis pubis to
properly measure the penis.

uinal and femoral areas

sk the patient to stand.
ell him to hold his breath and bear down while you inspect
ne inguinal and femoral areas for bulges or hernias (a loop of
owel that bulges through a muscle wall).

pation

is

se your thumb and forefinger to palpate the entire shaft of
ne penis. Note swelling, nodules, or indurations.
The penis should be somewhat firm.
The skin should be smooth and movable.

Testicles

- Assess the testicles' size, shape, and response to pressure.
  - A normal response is a deep visceral pain.
- Gently palpate both testicles between your thumb and first two fingers.
  - Testicles should be equal in size; feel firm, smooth, and rubbery; and move freely in the scrotal sac.
- If you note hard, irregular areas or lumps, transilluminate them. Do so by darkening the room and pressing the head of a flashlight against the scrotum, behind the lump. Transilluminate the other testicle and compare your findings.
  - The testicles and any lumps, masses, warts, or blood-filled areas will appear as opaque shadows.

Epididymides

- Palpate the epididymides.
  - They're usually located in the posterolateral area of the testicles.
  - They should be discrete, free from swelling and induration, nontender, and smooth.

Spermatic cords

- Palpate both spermatic cords, which are located above each testicle.
- Palpate from the base of the epididymis to the inguinal canal.
- If you feel swelling, irregularity, or nodules, transilluminate the problem area.
  - If serous fluid is present, you won't see a glow.

Inguinal area

- Assess the patient for a direct inguinal hernia:
  - First, place two fingers over each external inguinal ring.
  - Then ask the patient to bear down.
  - If a hernia is present, you'll feel a bulge.
- Assess for an indirect inguinal hernia:
  - First, examine the patient while he's standing.

alpating for an indirect inguinal hernia

Place your gloved fin-
er on the neck of the
crotum.
Insert it into the ingui-
al canal, as shown at
ght.
Ask the patient to bear
wn.
You'll feel a soft mass
your fingertip if the
tient has a hernia.

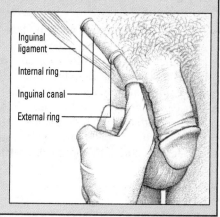

Inguinal ligament
Internal ring
Inguinal canal
External ring

Then examine him while he's in a supine position with his
nee flexed on the side you're examining.
Place your index finger on the neck of the scrotum.
Gently push upward into the inguinal canal.
After you've inserted your finger as far as possible, ask the
atient to bear down or cough.
A hernia feels like a mass of tissue that withdraws when it
eets the finger.

oral area

now that you can't palpate the femoral canal, but you can
stimate its location to help detect a femoral hernia.
lace your right index finger on the right femoral artery with
ur finger pointing toward the patient's head.
eep your other fingers together and close to the right index
ger.
est your middle finger on the femoral vein.
est your ring finger on the femoral canal.
ote tenderness or masses.

- Use your left hand and follow the same procedure to check the patient's left side.

Prostate gland

- Tell the patient that you need to place your finger in his rectum to examine his prostate gland.
- Explain that he'll feel some pressure or urgency to have a bowel movement during the examination.
- Have him stand and lean over the examination table.
- If he can't lean over the examination table, have him lie on left side with either his right knee and hip flexed or both of his knees drawn toward his chest.
- Inspect the skin of the perineal, anal, and posterior scrotal eas.
  – It should be smooth and unbroken, with no protruding masses.
- Lubricate the gloved index finger of your dominant hand.
- Insert your finger into the rectum.

Palpating the prostate gland

- Insert your lubricated, gloved index finger into the rectum.
- Palpate the prostate on the anterior rectal wall, just past the anorectal ring, as shown at right.

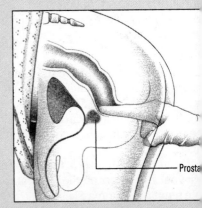

Prosta

Tell the patient to relax to ease the passage of the finger through the anal sphincter. If he has trouble relaxing, ask him to bear down as if he were having a bowel movement.

Palpate the prostate gland on the anterior rectal wall just past the anorectal ring with your finger pad.

- It should feel smooth and rubbery and should be about the size of a walnut.
- If the prostate gland protrudes into the rectal lumen, it's probably enlarged.
- Enlargement classifications range from grade 1 (protruding less than ⅜" [1 cm] into the rectal lumen) to grade 4 (protruding more than 1¼" [3.2 cm] into the rectal lumen).
- Ask the patient about tenderness and note any nodules.

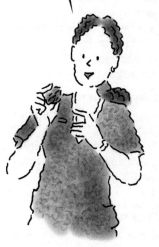

The prostate gland should be about the size of a walnut.

Abnormal findings

Urinary problems

Hematuria

- Presence of blood in the urine
- May turn the urine brown or bright red
- May indicate:
  - renal calculi
  - trauma to the urinary mucosa
  - urinary tract infection (UTI)
- May be a temporary condition after:
  - urethral catheterization
  - urinary tract or prostate surgery
- If present at the end of urination, signals a disorder of the:
  - bladder neck
  - prostate gland
  - urethra

Urinary frequency

- Abnormally frequent urination
- Symptom of:
  - benign prostatic hyperplasia (BPH)
  - prostate tumor (puts pressure on the bladder)
  - urethral stricture
  - UTI

Urinary urgency

- Intense and immediate desire to urinate
- Classic symptom of UTI

Urinary hesitancy

- Hesitancy at the beginning of the urine stream
- Most common in older patients who have enlarged prostate glands, which can partially obstruct the urethra

cturia

xcessive urination at night
common sign of renal or lower urinary tract disorders

Between the lines

valuating male genitourinary findings

gn or symptom and findings	Probable cause
nile lesions	
Fluid-filled vesicles on the glans penis, prepuce, or nile shaft Painful ulcers Tender inguinal lymph nodes Fever Malaise Dysuria	Genital herpes
Painless warts (tiny pink swellings that grow and come pedunculated) near the urethral meatus Lesions that have spread to the perineum and the rianal area Cauliflower-like appearance of multiple swellings	Genital warts
Sharply defined, slightly raised, scaling bilateral tches on the inner thigh or groin, scrotum, or penis Severe pruritus	Tinea cruris (jock itch)
rotal swelling	
wollen scrotum that's soft or unusually firm Bowel sounds that may be auscultated in the scro-	Hernia

(continued)

Evaluating male genitourinary findings *(continued)*

Sign or symptom and findings	Probable cau:
Scrotal swelling *(continued)* • Scrotal swelling that appeared gradually • Scrotum that's soft and cystic or firm and tense • Absence of pain • Round scrotal mass that isn't tender on palpation and glows when transilluminated	Hydrocele
• Scrotal swelling with sudden, severe pain • Unilateral elevation of the affected testicle • Nausea and vomiting	Testicular torsion
Penile discharge • Purulent or milky urethral discharge • Sudden fever and chills • Lower back pain • Myalgia • Perineal fullness • Arthralgia • Urinary frequency and urgency • Cloudy urine • Dysuria • Tense, boggy, very tender, warm prostate palpated during the digital rectal examination	Prostatitis
• Opaque, gray, yellowish, or blood-tinged discharge that's painless • Dysuria (eventually may become anuria)	Urethral neoplasm
• Scant or profuse urethral discharge that's thin and clear, mucoid, or thick and purulent • Urinary hesitancy, frequency, and urgency • Dysuria • Itching and burning around the meatus	Urethritis

valuating male genitourinary findings *(continued)*

gn or symptom and findings	Probable cause
inary hesitancy	BPH
Reduced caliber and force of urinary stream	
Perineal pain	
Feeling of incomplete voiding	
nability to stop urine stream	
Jrinary frequency	
Jrinary incontinence	
Bladder distention	
Jrinary frequency and dribbling	Prostate
Nocturia	cancer
Dysuria	
Bladder distention	
Perineal pain	
Constipation	
Hard, nodular prostate palpated on digital rectal amination	
Dysuria	UTI
Jrinary frequency and urgency	
Hematuria	
Cloudy urine	
Bladder spasms	
Costovertebral angle tenderness	
Suprapubic, low back, pelvic, or flank pain	
Jrethral discharge	

an result from:
BPH that causes significant urethral obstruction
diuretic medications
increased fluid intake
prostate cancer

Urinary incontinence
- Involuntary release of urine
- May be caused by:
  – BPH
  – prostate cancer
  – prostate infection

Reproductive system problems

Penile lesions
- Can vary in appearance
- May indicate penile cancer, especially if hard and nontende
  or nodule forms in the glans or inner lip of the prepuce

Penile discharge

Profuse, yellow discharge
- May be accompanied by other symptoms, such as urinary
  frequency, burning, and urgency
- Suggests gonococcal urethritis
- Without treatment, leads to inflammation of the prostate
  gland, epididymides, and periurethral glands

Copious, watery, purulent urethral discharge
- May indicate chlamydial infection

Bloody discharge
- May indicate infection or cancer

Paraphimosis
- Occurs when the prepuce is so tight that, when retracted, i
  gets caught behind the glans and can't be moved back into
  place
- Can cause edema
- May be prevented in uncircumcised men with frequent ret
  tion and cleaning of the prepuce (prevents excessive tightness, which in turn prevents the prepuce from closing off
  urinary meatus and constricting the glans)

Common male genital lesions

Penile cancer

- Painless, ulcerative lesion on the glans or prepuce
- Possibly accompanied by discharge

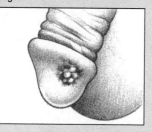

Genital warts

- Flesh-colored, soft, moist papillary growths that occur singly or in cauliflower-like clusters
- Barely visible or several inches in diameter

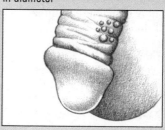

Genital herpes

- Painful, reddened group of small vesicles or blisters on the prepuce, shaft, or glans
- Eventually disappear but tend to recur

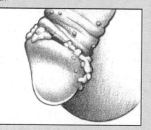

Syphilis

- Hard, round papule on the penis that may feel like a button when palpated and eventually erodes into an ulcer
- May cause swollen lymph nodes in the inguinal area

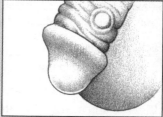

Displacement of the urethral meatus

- Can be one of two types:
  - epispadias—located on top of the penis
  - hydrospadias—located on the underside of the penis
- Congenital condition
- May contribute to infertility

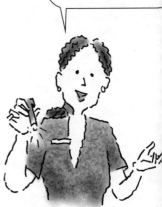

I'd like to shed some light on the subject for you; however, a testicular tumor can't be transilluminated.

Testicular tumor

- Painless scrotal nodule that can't be transilluminated
- Occurs most commonly in men ages 20 to 35
- Can grow and enlarge the testicle

Scrotal swelling

- Occurs when a condition affecting the testicles, epididymis or scrotal skin produces edema or a mass
- May be a sign of hydrocele (collection of fluid in the testicl
  - Associated with conditions that cause poor fluid reabsorp tion, such as cirrhosis, heart failure, and testicular tumors
  - Can be transilluminated
- May signal a hernia (a protrusion of an organ through an al normal opening in the muscle wall)

Prostate gland enlargement

- If the enlargement is smooth, firm, and symmetrical:
  - Indicates BPH, which typically starts after age 50
  - May be associated with nocturia, urinary hesitancy and f quency, and recurring UTIs

Types of hernias

Direct inguinal hernia
- Emerges from behind the external inguinal ring and protrudes through it
- Seldom descends into the scrotum
- Usually affects men older than age 40

Indirect inguinal hernia
- Most common type
- Occurs in men of all ages
- Can be palpated in the internal inguinal canal with its tip in or beyond the canal
- May descend into the scrotum

Femoral hernia
- Feels like a soft tumor below the inguinal ligament in the femoral area
- May be difficult to distinguish from a lymph node
- Uncommon in men

the enlargement if firm, warm, and extremely tender and swollen:
- Indicates acute prostatitis
- Is usually accompanied by fever because bacterial infection causes the condition

Prostate gland lesions
- Hard, irregular, fixed lesions that make the prostate feel asymmetrical
- Suggest prostate cancer
- May cause pain upon palpation
- Also cause urinary dysfunction
- In advanced stages, may have bone metastasis with back and leg pain

Priapism

- Considered a urologic emergency
- Persistent, painful erection that's unrelated to sexual excitation
  – Is usually accompanied by a severe, constant, dull aching in the penis
  – May last for several hours or days
- May lead to penile ischemia and thrombosis without prompt treatment
- May result from:
  – blood disorders (such as sickle cell anemia)
  – neoplasm
  – trauma
  – use of certain drugs

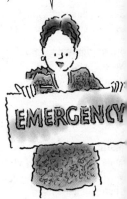

Priapism is a urologic emergency.

EMERGENCY

Erectile dysfunction

- Inability to achieve and maintain penile erection sufficient complete satisfactory sexual intercourse
- May affect ejaculation
- Varies from occasional and minimal to permanent and complete
- May result from:
  – age
  – drugs
  – fatigue
  – poor health
  – psychological, vascular, neurologic, or hormonal factors

Musculoskeletal system

14

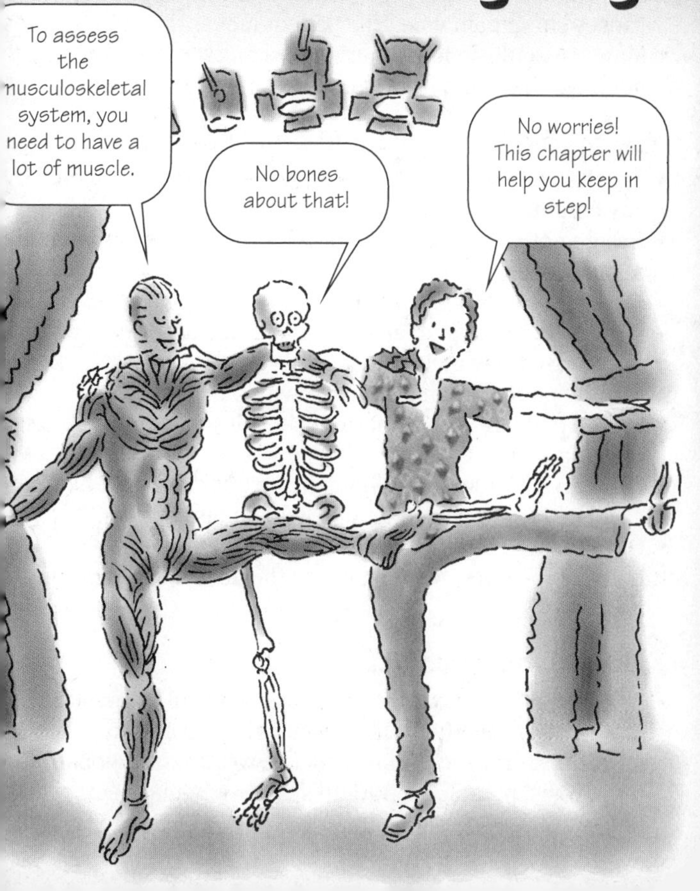

Health history

- Common musculoskeletal complaints include:
  – pain
  – swelling
  – stiffness
  – weakness
  – noticeable deformities.
- Deformities can also occur when a bone is fractured, which causes sharp pain when the patient moves the affected area
- Many musculoskeletal injuries are emergencies. You might not have time for a thorough assessment.

Asking about current and past health

- Are the patient's activities of daily living (ADLs) affected by any condition?
- Has he noticed grating sounds when he moves certain parts of his body?
- Does he use ice, heat, or other remedies to treat the problem
- Has he ever had gout, arthritis, tuberculosis, or cancer, which may cause bony metastasis?
- Has the patient been diagnosed with osteoporosis?
- Has he had a recent blunt or penetrating trauma? If so, how did it happen?
  – Did he suffer knee and hip injuries after being hit by a car?
  – Did he fall from a ladder and land on his coccyx?
- Does he use an assistive device, such as a cane, walker, or brace? If he does, watch him use the device to assess how he moves.

Asking about medications

- Ask the patient about the medications he takes regularly. Many drugs can affect the musculoskeletal system.
  – Corticosteroids can cause muscle weakness, myopathy, osteoporosis, pathologic fractures, and avascular necrosis of the heads of the femur and humerus.

Different strokes

Biocultural variations in bone density

Studies of bone density have shown that Black males have the densest bones.

– Black males also have a relatively low incidence of osteoporosis, a bone disorder characterized by a decrease in bone mass that leaves bones porous, brittle, and prone to fractures.

White patients' bone density levels are typically lower than the density levels of Black patients but higher than those of Chinese, Japanese, and Inuit patients.

– Potassium-depleting diuretics can cause muscle cramping and weakness.

Asking about lifestyle

Ask about the patient's job, hobbies, and personal habits.

– Working at a computer, knitting, playing football or tennis, or doing construction work can cause repetitive stress injuries or injure the musculoskeletal system in other ways.

– Carrying a heavy knapsack or purse can cause injury or increase muscle size.

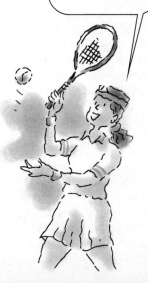

Activities such as tennis can cause repetitive stress injuries.

Physical assessment

- Assessment will help uncover musculoskeletal abnormalitie and evaluate the patient's ability to perform ADLs.
- Assess the central nervous and musculoskeletal systems together.
- Use inspection and palpation to test the major bones, joints and muscles.
- Bring a tape measure — the only special equipment needed.
- Perform a complete examination if the patient has generalized symptoms such as aching in several joints.
- Perform an abbreviated examination if he has pain in only one body area.
- Before starting your assessment, have the patient undress down to his underwear and then put on a hospital gown.
- Make sure the room is warm.
- Explain each procedure as you perform it.
- Begin your examination with a general observation of the pa tient.
- Then systematically assess the whole body, working from head to toe and from proximal to distal structures.
- Because muscles and joints are interdependent, interpret these findings together.
- Note the size and shape of joints, limbs, and body regions.
- Inspect and palpate the skin and tissues around the joint, limbs, and body regions.
- Have the patient perform active range-of-motion (ROM) exe cises (joint movements the patient can do without assistance), if possible.
- If he can't perform active ROM exercises, perform passive ROM exercises (exercises that don't require the patient to e ert effort).
  - Support the joint firmly on either side.
  - Move the joint gently to avoid causing pain or spasm.
  - Never force movement.
- Observe how the patient stands and moves.

Watch him walk into the room or, if he's inside the room, ask him to walk to the door, turn around, and walk back.

– The torso should sway only slightly.
– Arms should swing naturally at his sides.
– Gait should be even.
– Posture should be erect.
– Each foot should flatten and bear his weight completely.
– Toes should flex as he pushes off with his foot.
– In midswing, his foot should clear the floor and pass the other leg.
– If you note a child with a waddling, ducklike gait (an indication of muscular dystrophy), check for a positive Gowers' sign, which indicates pelvic muscle weakness.

Identifying Gowers' sign

Place the patient in the supine position.

Ask him to rise.

A positive sign for Gowers' — the patient's inability to lift his trunk without using his hands and arms to brace and push — indicates pelvic muscle weakness, which occurs in muscular dystrophy and spinal muscle atrophy.

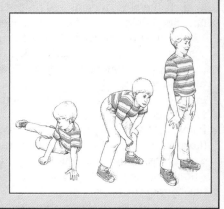

Assessing the bones and joints

Perform a head-to-toe evaluation of your patient's bones and joints using inspection and palpation.

Perform ROM exercises to help you determine whether the joints are healthy.

– Never force movement.
– Ask the patient to tell you when he experiences pain.
– Watch his facial expression for signs of pain or discomfort.

Head, jaw, and neck

- Inspect the patient's face for swelling, symmetry, and evidence of trauma.
  – The mandible should be in the midline, not shifted to the right or left.
- Evaluate the patient's ROM in the temporomandibular joint (TMJ).
  – Place the tips of your first two or three fingers in front of the middle of the ear.
  – Ask the patient to open and close his mouth.
  – Place your fingers into the depressed area over the joint.
  – Note the motion of the mandible; the patient should be able to open and close the jaw and protract and retract the mandible easily, without pain or tenderness.
  – If you hear or palpate a click as the patient's mouth opens, suspect an improperly aligned jaw.
  – TMJ dysfunction may also lead to swelling of the area, crepitus (abnormal grating sound), or pain.
- Inspect the front, back, and sides of the patient's neck, noting muscle asymmetry or masses.
- Palpate the spinous processes of the cervical vertebrae and the areas above each clavicle (supraclavicular fossae) for tenderness, swelling, or nodules.
  – Stand facing the patient with your hands placed lightly on the sides of the neck.
  – Ask him to turn his head from side to side, flex his neck forward, and then extend it backward.
  – Feel for any lumps or tender areas.
  – Listen and palpate for crepitus as the patient moves his neck.
- Check ROM in the neck.

- Ask the patient to try touching his right ear to his right shoulder and his left ear to his left shoulder; typical ROM is 40 degrees on each side.
- Ask him to touch his chin to his chest and then to point his chin toward the ceiling; the neck should flex forward 45 degrees and extend backward 55 degrees.
- Ask the patient to turn his head to each side without moving his trunk to assess rotation; his chin should be parallel to his shoulders.
- Ask him to move his head in a circle; a normal rotation is 70 degrees.

ine

Ask the patient to remove his hospital gown so you can observe his spine.

Check his spinal curvature as he stands in profile.
- The spine should have a reverse "S" shape.

Observe the spine posteriorly.
- It should be in midline position, without deviation to either side.
- Lateral deviation suggests scoliosis.
- One shoulder may be lower than the other.

To assess for scoliosis, ask the patient to bend at the waist, which makes deformities more apparent.
- Normally, the spine remains at midline.

Assess the range of spinal movement.
- Ask the patient to straighten up.
- Use a measuring tape to determine the distance from the nape of his neck to his waist.
- Ask him to bend forward at the waist.
- Continue to hold the tape at his neck, letting slip through your fingers slightly to accomodate the increased distance as the spine lexes.

> The patient's spine shouldn't deviate to the right or left side.

Kyphosis and lordosis

Kyphosis
• The thoracic curve is abnormally rounded, as shown below.

Lordosis
• The lumbar spine is abnormally concave, as shown below.
• Lordosis (as well as a waddling gait) is normal in pregnant women and young children.

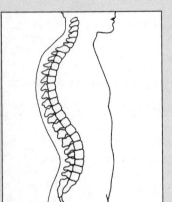

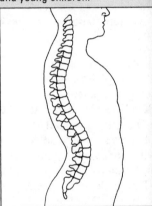

– The length of the spine from neck to waist usually increases by at least 2″ (5.1 cm) when the patient bends forward; if it doesn't, the patient's mobility may be impaired, and you'll need to assess him further.
• Palpate the spinal processes and the areas lateral to the spine
  – Have the patient bend at the waist and let his arms hang loosely at his sides.
  – Palpate the spine with your fingertips.
  – Repeat the palpation using the side of your hand, lightly striking the areas lateral to the spine.
  – Note tenderness, swelling, or spasm.

Testing for scoliosis

Ask the patient to
remove his shirt and
stand as straight as pos-
sible with his back to
you. Look for:
– uneven shoulder
height and shoulder
blade prominence
– unequal distance
between the arms and
the body
– asymmetrical waist-
line
– uneven hip height
– sideways lean.
Then ask the patient to
bend forward, keeping
his head down and palms
together. Look for:
– asymmetrical thoracic spine or prominent rib cage (rib hump) on
either side
– asymmetrical waistline.

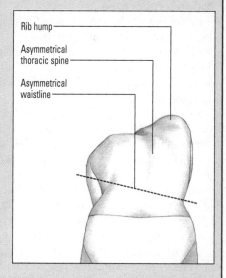

Rib hump

Asymmetrical
thoracic spine

Asymmetrical
waistline

Shoulders and elbows

Observe the patient's shoulders and note any asymmetry,
muscle atrophy, or deformity.
- Swelling or loss of the normal rounded shape could mean
that one or more bones are dislocated or out of alignment.
- If the patient's reason for seeking care is shoulder pain, the
problem may not have originated in the shoulder. Shoulder
pain may be referred from other sources and may be due to a
heart attack or ruptured ectopic pregnancy.
Palpate the shoulders with the palmar surfaces of your fingers.
- Locate bony landmarks.

- Note crepitus or tenderness.
- Palpate the shoulder muscles for firmness and symmetry using your entire hand.
- Palpate the elbow and the ulna for subcutaneous nodules that occur with rheumatoid arthritis.
- Assess shoulder rotation if the patient's shoulders don't appear to be dislocated.
  - Start with the patient's arm in the neutral position (straight at his side).
  - Ask him to lift his arm straight up from his side to shoulder level. Then tell him to bend his elbow horizontally until his forearm is at a 90-degree angle to his upper arm. His arm should be parallel to the floor, and his fingers should be extended with palms down.
  - To assess external rotation, have him bring his forearm up until his fingers point toward the ceiling.
  - To assess internal rotation, have him lower his forearm until his fingers point toward the floor.
  - A normal ROM is 90 degrees in each direction.
- To assess flexion and extension, ask the patient to put his arms at his side, in the neutral position.
- To assess flexion, ask him to move his arm forward over his head, as if reaching for the sky.
  - Full flexion is 180 degrees.
- To assess extension, have him move his arm from the neutral position back as far as possible.
  - A normal extension ranges from 30 to 50 degrees.
- To assess abduction, ask the patient to move his arm from the neutral position laterally as far as possible.
  - Normal ROM is 180 degrees.
- To assess adduction, have the patient move his arm from the neutral position across the front of his body as far as possible.
  - Normal ROM is 50 degrees.
- Assess the elbows for flexion and extension.
  - Have the patient rest his arm at his side.

- Ask him to flex his elbow from this position and then extend it.
- Normal ROM is 90 degrees for both flexion and extension.

To assess supination and pronation of the elbow, have the patient place the side of his hand on a flat surface with the thumb on top.
- Ask him to rotate his palm down toward the table for pronation and upward for supination.
- Normal angle of elbow rotation is 90 degrees in each direction.

Wrists and hands

Inspect the patient's wrists and hands for contour, and compare them for symmetry.
- Check for nodules, redness, swelling, deformities, and webbing between his fingers.

Use your thumb and index finger to palpate both wrists and each finger joint.
- Ask the patient about tenderness and note nodules, or bogginess.
- To avoid causing pain, be especially gentle with elderly patients and those with arthritis.

Assess ROM in the wrists.
- Ask the patient to rotate each wrist by moving his entire hand — first laterally and then medially — as if he's waxing a car.

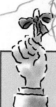

Memory jogger

Here's an easy way to keep adduction and abduction straight:

Adduction is moving a limb toward the body's midline. Think of it as **adding** two things together.

Abduction is moving a limb away from the body's midline. Think of it as taking something away, as in **abducting,** or kidnapping.

Be gentle when assessing the wrists and hands of elderly patients and those with arthritis.

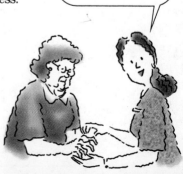

– Normal ROM is 55 degrees laterally and 20 degrees medial

- Observe the wrist while the patient extends his fingers up to ward the ceiling and down toward the floor, as if he's flappi his hand.

  – Normal wrist extension is 70 degrees.

  – Normal wrist flexion is 90 degrees.

  – If these movements cause the patient pain or numbness, h may have carpal tunnel syndrome.

Testing for carpal tunnel syndrome

Tinel's sign

- Lightly percuss the transverse carpal ligament over the median nerve where the patient's palm and wrist meet.
- If this action produces discomfort, such as numbness and tingling shooting into the palm and finger, the patient has Tinel's sign and may have carpal tunnel syndrome.

Phalen's maneuver

- If flexing the patient's wrist for about 30 seconds causes pain or numbness in his hand or fingers, he has a positive Phalen's sign.
- The more severe the carpal tunnel syndrome, the more rapidly the symptoms develop.

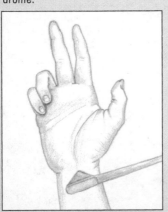

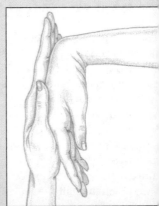

Assess extension and flexion of the metacarpophalangeal joints.

- Ask the patient to keep his wrist still and move only his fingers — first up toward the ceiling and then down toward the floor.
- Normal extension is 30 degrees.
- Normal flexion is 90 degrees.
- Ask the patient to touch the thumb on one hand to the little finger of the same hand.
- He should be able to fold or flex his thumb across the palm of his hand so that it touches or points toward the base of his little finger.

Assess flexion of all of the fingers.

- Ask the patient to form a fist.
- Have him spread his fingers apart to demonstrate abduction and draw them back together to demonstrate adduction.

Take measurements if you suspect that one arm is longer than the other.

- Put one end of the measuring tape at the acromial process of the shoulder and the other end on the tip of the middle finger.
- Drape the tape over the outer elbow.
- The difference between the left and right extremities should be no more than ⅜″ (1 cm).

Hips and knees

Inspect the hip area for contour and symmetry.

Inspect the position of the patient's knees, noting whether he's:

- bowlegged (with knees that point out).
- knock-kneed (with knees that turn in).

Watch the patient walk.

Palpate each of his hips over the iliac crest and trochanteric area for tenderness or instability.

Palpate both knees.

- Knees should feel smooth.

– Tissues should feel solid.
– The bulge sign indicates excess fluid in the joint.

Assessing for the bulge sign

• Ask the patient to lie down so that you can palpate his knee.
• Give the medial side of his knee two to four firm strokes, as shown below, to displace excess fluid.

• Tap the lateral aspect of the knee while checking for a fluid wave on the medial aspect (as shown below).

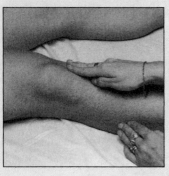
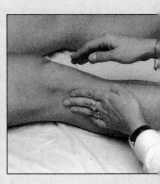

• Assess ROM in the hip with the patient in a supine position
• To assess hip flexion:
    – Place your hand under the patient's lower back.
    – Have the patient bend one knee and pull it toward his abdomen and chest as far as possible.
    – You'll feel the patient's back touch your hand as the norm lumbar lordosis of the spine flattens.
    – As the patient flexes his knee, the opposite hip and thigh should remain flat on the bed.
    – Repeat these steps on the opposite side.
• To assess hip abduction:

– Stand alongside the patient and press down on the superior iliac spine of the opposite hip with one hand to stabilize the pelvis.

– With your other hand, hold the patient's leg by the ankle.

– Gently abduct the hip until you feel the iliac spine move.

– Movement of the iliac spine indicates the limit of hip abduction.

– While still stabilizing the pelvis, move the patient's ankle medially across his body to assess hip adduction.

– Repeat these steps on the other side.

– Normal ROM is about 45 degrees for abduction and 30 degrees for adduction.

To assess hip extension:

– Have the patient lie prone (face down).

– Gently extend the thigh upward.

– Repeat these steps on the other thigh.

To assess internal and external rotation of the hip:

– Ask the patient to lift one leg up.

– Keeping his knee straight, turn his leg and foot medially and laterally.

– Normal ROM for internal rotation is 40 degrees.

– Normal ROM for external rotation is 45 degrees.

Assess ROM in the knees.

– If the patient is standing, ask him to bend one knee as if trying to touch his heel to his buttocks.

– Normal ROM for flexion is 120 to 130 degrees.

– If the patient is lying down, have him draw his knee up to his chest; his calf should touch his thigh.

– Knee extension returns the knee to a neutral position of 0 degrees.

– Some knees may normally be hyperextended 15 degrees.

– If the patient can't extend his leg fully or if his knee pops audibly and painfully, consider the response abnormal.

– Pronounced crepitus may signal a degenerative disease of the knee.

– Sudden buckling may indicate a ligament injury.

Ankles and feet

- Inspect the ankles and feet for swelling, redness, nodules, ar other deformities.
- Check the arch of the foot and look for toe deformities.
- Note:
  - bunions, calluses, and corns
  - edema
  - hair loss
  - ingrown toenails
  - plantar warts
  - trophic ulcers
  - unusual pigmentation.
- Use your fingertips to palpate the patient's bony and muscular structures of his ankles and feet.
- Palpate each toe joint by compressing it with your thumb ar fingers.
- Examine the ankle.
  - Have the patient sit in a chair or on the side of a bed.
  - To test plantar flexion, ask him to point his toes toward the floor.
  - To test dorsiflexion, ask him to point his toes toward the ceiling.
  - Normal ROM for plantar flexion is about 45 degrees.
  - Normal ROM for dorsiflexion is about 20 degrees.
  - Ask the patient to demonstrate inversion by turning his fee inward, and eversion by turning his feet outward.
  - Normal ROM for inversion is 45 degrees.
  - Normal ROM for eversion is 30 degrees.
- Assess the metatarsophalangeal joints.
  - Ask the patient to flex his toes and then straighten them.
- Take measurements if one leg appears longer than the other.
  - Put one end of the tape at the medial malleolus at the ankle and the other end at the anterior iliac spine.
  - Cross the tape over the medial side of the knee.
  - A difference of more than $\frac{3}{8}''$ (1 cm) is abnormal.

ssessing the muscles

Inspect the patient's major muscle groups for tone, strength, and symmetry.

---

esting muscle strength

iceps strength
ull down on the flexor surface of
he patient's forearm as he resists.

Ankle strength: Plantar flexion
Have the patient push his foot
down against your resistance.

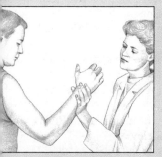

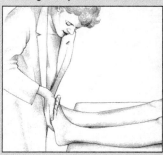

riceps strength
ave the patient try to straighten
is arm as you push upward
gainst the extensor surface of
is forearm.

Ankle strength: Dorsiflexion
Have the patient pull his foot up
as you try to hold it down.

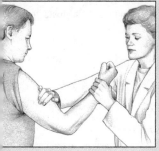

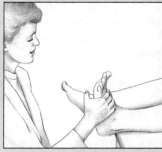

Grading muscle strength

Grade	Classification	Description
5/5	Normal	The patient can move the joint through full ROM and against gravity with full resistance.
4/5	Good	The patient can complete ROM tests against gravity with moderate resistance.
3/5	Fair	The patient can complete ROM tests against gravity only.
2/5	Poor	The patient can complete full ROM tests with gravity eliminated (passive motion).
1/5	Trace	The patient's attempt at muscle contraction is palpable but he doesn't have joint movement.
0/5	Zero	The patient's attempt shows no evidence of muscle contraction.

- If a muscle appears atrophied or hypertrophied:
  - Measure the muscle on each side of the body by wrapping tape measure around the largest circumference of the musc
  - Compare the two measurements.
- Other abnormalities of muscle appearance include:
  - contracture
  - abnormal movements, such as spasms, tics, tremors, and fasciculations.
- To test muscle tone (muscular resistance to passive stretching) in the arm:
  - Move the patient's shoulders through passive ROM exercises. You should feel a slight resistance.
  - Then let his arm drop. It should fall easily to his side.

To test leg muscle tone:
- Put the patient's hip through passive ROM exercises.
- Let the leg fall to the examination table or bed. Like the arm, the leg should fall easily.

Observe the patient's gait and movements to form an idea of his general muscle strength.
- Grade muscle strength on a scale of 0 to 5, with 0 representing no strength and 5 representing maximum strength.
- Document the results as a fraction, with the score as the numerator and maximum strength as the denominator.

To test specific muscle groups:
- Ask the patient to move the muscles while you apply resistance.
- Compare the contralateral muscle groups.

Shoulder, arm, wrist, and hand strength

Test the strength of the patient's shoulder girdle by asking him to extend his arms with the palms up and hold the position for 30 seconds.
- If he can't lift both arms equally and keep his palms up, or if one arm drifts down, he probably has shoulder girdle weakness on that side.
- If he passes the first part of the test, gauge his strength by placing your hands on his arms and applying downward pressure as he resists you.
- Have the patient hold his arm in front of him with the elbow bent.

Testing handgrip strength

Face the patient.
Extend the first and second fingers of your hands.
Ask him to grasp your fingers and squeeze.
Don't extend fingers with rings on them because a strong handgrip on those fingers can be painful.

- To test bicep strength, pull down on the flexor surface of hi
  forearm as he resists.
- To test triceps strength, have him try to straighten his arm a
  you push upward against the extensor surface of his forearm
- Assess the strength of the patient's flexed wrist by pushing
  against it.
- Test the strength of the extended wrist by pushing down on
- Test the strength of finger abduction, thumb opposition, an
  handgrip the same way.

Leg strength

- Ask the patient to lie in a supine position on the examinatic
  table or bed.
  – Have him lift both legs at the same time.
  – Note whether he lifts both legs at the same time and to the
  same distance.
- Test quadriceps strength.
  – Have the patient lower his legs and raise
  them again while you press down on his
  anterior thighs.
- Ask the patient to flex his knees and put
  his feet flat on the bed.
- Assess lower-leg
  strength.
  – Pull the patient's lower
  leg forward as he resists.
  – Then push the leg
  backward as he extends
  his knee.
- Assess ankle strength.
  – Have the patient push
  his foot down against
  your resistance.
  – Then ask him to pull
  his foot up as you try to
  hold it down.

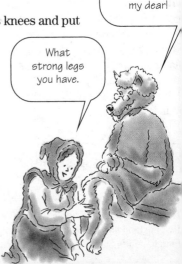

The better to walk with, my dear!

What strong legs you have.

normal findings

m pain

- ocated anywhere from the hand to the shoulder
- Jsually results from musculoskeletal disorders
- Can also stem from neurovascular or cardiovascular disorders
- n some cases, may be referred pain from:
  - abdomen
  - chest
  - neck

epitus

bnormal crunching or grating
eard or felt when a joint with
oughened articular surfaces
noves
Occurs in patients with:
- rheumatoid arthritis
- osteoarthritis
- broken pieces of bone that rub
gether

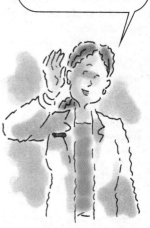

Hear a crunching
sound when a joint
moves? That's crepitus.

otdrop

lantar flexion of the foot with
ne toes bent toward the instep
esults from weakness or paraly-
s of the dorsiflexor muscles of the foot and ankle
ign of certain peripheral nerve or motor neuron disorders
lay stem from prolonged immobility when these circum-
ances produce shortening of the Achilles tendon:
- inadequate support
- improper positioning
- infrequent passive exercise

(Text continues on page 273.)

Between the lines

Evaluating musculoskeletal findings

Sign or symptom and findings	Probable cause
Arm pain • Radiates through the patient's arm • Crepitus felt and heard • Deformity if bones are misaligned • Impaired distal circulation • Local ecchymosis and edema • Paresthesia • Worsens with movement	Fracture
• Left arm • Deep and crushing chest pain • Apprehension • Diaphoresis • Dyspnea • Pallor • Weakness	Myocardial infarction
• Severe with passive muscle stretching • Decreased reflex response • Edema • Impaired distal circulation • Muscle weakness • Paralysis and no pulse (ominous signs) • Paresthesia	Compartment syndrome

Evaluating musculoskeletal findings *(continued)*

Sign or symptom and findings	Probable cause
Leg pain	
Severe, acute leg pain, particularly with movement	Fracture
Deformity, crepitus, and muscle spasms	
Ecchymosis and edema	
Impaired neurovascular status distal to injury	
Inability of leg to bear weight	
Shooting, aching, or tingling sensation that radiates down the leg	Sciatica
Difficulty moving from a sitting to a standing position	
Exacerbated by activity and relieved by rest	
Limping	
Discomfort ranging from calf tenderness to severe pain	Thrombophlebitis
Edema and a feeling of heaviness in the affected leg	
Fever, chills, malaise, and muscle cramps	
Positive Homans' sign	
Warmth	
Muscle spasm	
With intermittent claudication	Arterial occlusive disease
Decreased sensation	
Dry or scaling skin	
Edema	
Hair loss	
Loss of peripheral pulses	
Pallor or cyanosis	
Ulcerations	

(continued)

Evaluating musculoskeletal findings *(continued)*

Sign or symptom and findings	Probable cause
Muscle spasm *(continued)* • Localized and accompanied by pain • Bony crepitation • Limited mobility • Swelling	Fracture
• Tetany (muscle cramps and twitching, carpopedal and facial muscle spasms, and seizures) • Cardiac arrhythmias • Choreiform movements • Fatigue • Hyperactive deep tendon reflexes • Palpitations • Paresthesia of the lips, fingers, and toes • Positive Chvostek's and Trousseau's signs	Hypocalcemia
Muscle weakness • Unilateral or bilateral in the arms, legs, face, or tongue • Aphasia • Bowel and bladder dysfunction • Dysarthria • Paresthesia or sensory loss • Vision disturbances	Stroke
• Muscle weakness, disuse, and possible atrophy • Altered level of consciousness • Diminished reflexes • Personality changes • Sensory changes • Severe low back pain, possibly radiating to the buttocks, legs, and feet (usually unilateral)	Herniated disk

valuating musculoskeletal findings *(continued)*

gn or symptom and findings	**Probable cause**
uscle weakness *(continued)* In one or more limbs, possibly leading to atrophy, asticity, and contractures Diplopia, blurred vision, or vision loss Hyperactive deep tendon reflexes Incoordination Intention tremors Paresthesia or sensory loss	Multiple sclerosis

g pain

Commonly indicates a musculoskeletal disorder
Can result from more serious vascular
r neurologic disorders
May occur suddenly or gradually
May be localized or affect the entire
eg
May be constant or intermittent
May feel a burning, dull, sharp,
hooting, or tingling sensation

uscle atrophy

Results from denervation or pro-
onged muscle disuse
Occurs because muscle fibers lose
ulk and length, which produces:
 visible loss of muscle size and
ontour
 apparent emaciation or deformi-
y in the area deprived of regular
xercise

> With muscle atrophy, muscle fibers lose bulk and length.

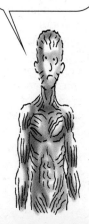

- Usually results from:
  - neuromuscular disease
  - injury
- May stem from:
  - metabolic and endocrine disorders
  - prolonged immobility
- Occurs with aging

Muscle spasms

- Strong, painful contractions
- Can occur in virtually any muscle
- Most common in the calf and foot
- Typically occur:
  - after exercise
  - during pregnancy
  - from simple muscle fatigue
- May develop:
  - in electrolyte imbalances and neuromuscular disorders
  - as an effect of certain drugs

Muscle weakness

- Can result from a malfunction in:
  - myoneural junctions
  - nerve roots
  - peripheral nerves
  - the brain stem
  - the cerebral hemispheres
  - the muscle itself
  - the spinal cord
- May be detected by observing and measuring the strength of an individual muscle or muscle group
- May be reported to you by the patient

Muscle rigidity

Indicates increased muscle tone

Possibly caused by upper motor neuron lesions, such as those resulting from a stroke

Muscle flaccidity

May result from a lower motor neuron lesion

Traumatic injuries

The cause of most musculoskeletal emergencies

Include:

- amputations
- crush injuries
- dislocations
- fractures
- serious lacerations

The 5 P's of musculoskeletal injury

Pain

Ask the patient whether he feels pain.

If he feels pain, assess its location, severity, and quality.

Paresthesia

Touch the injured area with the tip of an open safety pin.

Abnormal sensation or loss of sensation indicates neurovascular involvement.

Paralysis

Assess whether the patient can move the affected area.

• If he can't move the area, he might have nerve or tendon damage.

Pallor

• Paleness, discoloration, and coolness on the injured side may indicate neurovascular compromise.

Pulse

• Check all pulses distal to the injury site.

• If a pulse is decreased or absent, blood supply to the area is reduced.

Heberden's and Bouchard's nodes

- Hard nodes that develop on the distal and proximal joints of the fingers in patients with osteoarthritis
- May be accompanied by:
  - contracture
  - crepitus
  - joint swelling
  - limited movement
  - pain
- May affect gait if knees and hips are involved

Heberden's and Bouchard's nodes

Heberden's nodes
- Appear on the distal interphalangeal joints
- Usually hard and painless
- Bony and cartilaginous enlargements
- Typically occur in middle-aged and elderly patients with osteoarthritis

Bouchard's nodes
- Are similar to Heberden's node but are less common
- Appear on the proximal interphalangeal joints

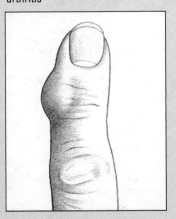
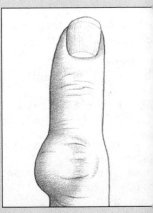

Neurologic system

15

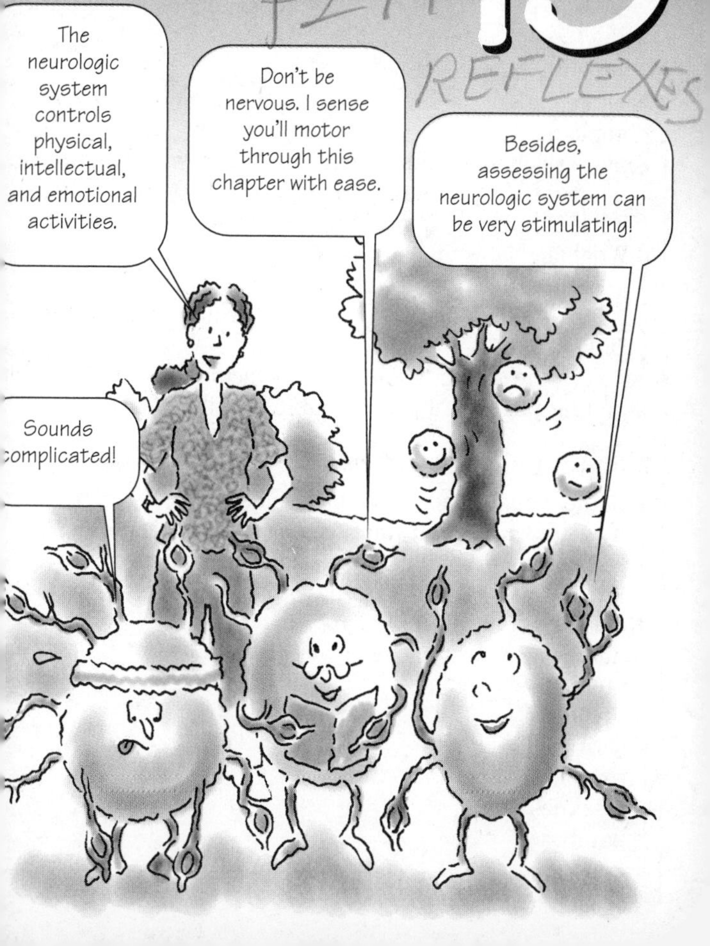

Health history

- Common complaints about the neurologic system include:
  - changes in level of consciousness (LOC)
  - confusion
  - disturbances in balance or gait
  - dizziness
  - faintness
  - headache
  - impaired mental status.
- Use the patient's own words when documenting the chief complaint.
- Ask these questions about each of the patient's symptoms:
  - When did the problem start and how often does it occur?
  - What factors precipitate and exacerbate the problem?
  - What alleviates the problem?
  - Do other symptoms accompany this problem?
  - Has the patient had adverse effects from treatment for the problem?
- Also ask the patient about other aspects of his current health, about his past health, and about his family history.

Asking about current health

- Ask the patient whether he has headaches.
  - If so, how often and what seems to bring them on?
  - Does light bother his eyes during a headache?
  - What other symptoms occur with a headache?
- Does the patient have:
  - dizziness?
  - numbness?
  - tingling?
  - seizures?
  - tremors?
  - weakness?
  - paralysis?

Does he have problems with:
- any of his senses?
- walking?
- keeping his balance?
- swallowing?
- urinating?

Does he ever have trouble speaking or understanding what people say?

Does he have trouble reading or writing? If so, how much does this interfere with his daily activities?

Some neurologic changes, such as decreased reflexes, hearing, and vision, are a normal part of aging.

How does he rate his memory and ability to concentrate?

Ask about the patient's medication regimen. Some drugs can affect the neurologic system, especially in elderly patients. Determine whether the changes are asymmetric, indicating a pathologic condition, and whether abnormalities need further investigation.

Asking about past health

Ask the patient about his past health conditions, including:
- major illnesses such as cancer

Aging and the neurologic system

Because neurons undergo various degenerative changes, aging can lead to:
- decreased agility
- decreased acuity of the senses, such as hearing, vision, taste, and smell
- decreased vibratory sense in the ankles
- development of muscle tremors, commonly in the head and hands
- diminished reflexes
- slowed reaction time.

– recurrent minor illnesses such as ear infections
– accidents or injuries
– surgical procedures
– allergies.

Asking about family history

• Ask about the patient's family history.
– Some genetic diseases are degenerative; others cause muscle weakness.
– Incidence of seizures is higher in patients whose family history shows idiopathic epilepsy.
– More than one-half of patients with migraine headaches have a family history of the disorder.

Physical assessment

Patients who suffer from diseases of other body systems can develop neurologic impairments related to their diseases.
- A patient who has heart surgery may also suffer a stroke. Daily nursing care may routinely include some neurologic status tests.
A full neurologic examination is so long and detailed that you will rarely complete an entire exam.
If your initial screening examination suggests a neurologic problem, you may want to perform a detailed assessment. Begin with the highest levels of neurologic function and work down to the lowest, covering these five areas:
- cranial nerve function
- mental status and speech
- motor function
- reflexes
- sensory function.

Assessing mental status and speech

Mental status assessment begins when you talk to the patient during the health history.
Talking with a patient helps you assess:
- orientation
- LOC
- ability to formulate and produce speech
- what to look for during your physical assessment.
Ask questions that require more than "yes" or "no" answers.

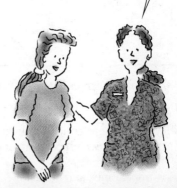

Simply talking with your patient can help you assess mental status and speech.

A quick check of mental status

To quickly screen patients for disordered thought processes, ask the questions below. An incorrect answer to any question may indicate the need for a complete mental status examination. Make sure you know the correct answers before asking the questions.

Question	Function screened
What's your name?	Orientation to person
What's your mother's name?	Orientation to other people
What year is it?	Orientation to time
Where are you now?	Orientation to place
How old are you?	Memory
Where were you born?	Remote memory
What did you have for breakfast?	Recent memory
Who's currently president of the United States?	General knowledge
Can you count backward from 20 to 1?	Attention span and calculation skills

- Perform a screening examination if you have doubts about a patient's mental status.
- If the patient talks about his confusion or memory problems, you'll want to concentrate on the mental status part of the examination, which consists of checking:
  - LOC
  - appearance and behavior

- speech
- cognitive function
- constructional ability.

Level of consciousness

A change in the patient's LOC is the earliest and most sensitive indicator that neurologic status has changed.

Clearly describe the patient's response to various stimuli using these terms:

- Alert — follows commands and responds completely and appropriately to stimuli
- Lethargic — is drowsy; has delayed responses to verbal stimuli; may drift off to sleep during examination
- Stuporous — requires vigorous stimulation for a response
- Comatose — doesn't respond appropriately to verbal or painful stimuli; can't follow commands or communicate verbally.

Observe the patient's LOC.

- Is he alert, or is he falling asleep?
- Can he focus his attention and maintain it, for example, or is he easily distracted?

If you need to use a stronger stimulus than your voice, record:

- what stimulus you use
- how strong the stimulus needs to be to get a response from the patient.

Use the Glasgow Coma Scale as a way to objectively assess the patient's LOC.

Appearance and behavior

Note how the patient behaves, dresses, and grooms himself. Are his appearance and behavior appropriate?

Is his personal hygiene poor? If you believe it is, discuss your findings with the family to determine whether this behavior is a change. Even subtle changes in a patient's behavior can sig-

Using the Glasgow Coma Scale

- Test the patient's ability to respond to verbal, motor, and sensory stimulation; grade his responses according to the scale below.
- A patient's score will total 15 points if he's:
  - able to follow simple commands
  - alert
  - oriented to time, place, and person.
- A lower score in one or more categories may signal an impending neurologic crisis.
- A total score of 7 or less indicates severe neurologic damage.

Test	Score	Patient's response
Eye-opening response		
Spontaneously	4	Opens eyes spontaneously
To speech	3	Opens eyes when told to
To pain	2	Opens eyes only on painful stimulus
None	1	Doesn't open eyes in response to stimulus
Motor response		
Obeys	6	Shows two fingers when asked
Localizes	5	Reaches toward painful stimulus and tries to remove it
Withdraws	4	Moves away from painful stimulus
Abnormal flexion	3	Assumes a decorticate posture
Abnormal extension	2	Assumes a decerebrate posture
None	1	No response; just lies flaccid, which is an ominous sign

Using the Glasgow Coma Scale (continued)

Test	Score	Patient's response
Verbal response		
Oriented	5	Reports current date
Confused	4	Reports incorrect year
Inappropriate words	3	Replies randomly with incorrect word
Incomprehensible	2	Moans or screams
None	1	No response
Total score		

nal a new onset of a chronic disease or a more acute change that involves the frontal lobe.

Speech

Listen carefully to determine how well the patient expresses himself.
– Is his speech fluent or fragmented?
– Note the pace, volume, clarity, and spontaneity of his speech.
To assess for dysarthria (difficulty forming words), ask him to repeat the phrase "no ifs, ands, or buts."
Assess comprehension by determining his ability to follow instructions and cooperate with your examination.

Cognitive function

Assessing the patient's cognitive function involves testing:
– memory
– orientation
– attention span
– calculation ability
– thought content
– abstract thinking

- judgment
- insight
- emotional status.
- Use the questions previously outlined in *A quick check of mental status* to test your patient's orientation, memory, and attention span.
  - Orientation to time is usually disrupted first.
  - Orientation to person is usually disrupted last.
- Consider the patient's environment and physical condition when assessing orientation.
  - An elderly patient admitted to the hospital for several days may not be oriented to time, especially if he has been bedridden.
  - When the person is intubated and can't speak, ask questions that require only a nod, such as "Do you know you're in the hospital?" and "Are we in Pennsylvania?"

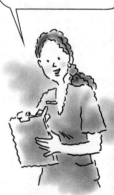

A patient's orientation to time is usually disrupted before his orientation to person is.

- Short-term memory is commonly affected first in patients with neurologic disease.
  - A patient with an intact short-term memory can generally repeat five to seven nonconsecutive numbers right away and again 10 minutes later.
- When testing attention span and calculation skills, keep in mind that lack of mathematical ability and anxiety can affect the patient's performance.
  - If he has difficulty with numerical computation, ask him to spell the word "world" backward.
  - While he's completing these tests, note his ability to pay attention.

Assess thought content by evaluating the clarity and cohesiveness of the patient's ideas.
– Is his conversation smooth, with logical transitions between ideas?
– Does he have hallucinations (sensory perceptions that lack appropriate stimuli) or delusions (beliefs not supported by reality)?
– Disordered thought patterns may indicate delirium or psychosis.

Test the patient's ability to think abstractly by asking him to interpret a common proverb such as "A stitch in time saves nine."
– A patient with dementia may interpret this proverb literally.
– If the patient's primary language isn't English, he'll probably have difficulty interpreting the proverb.
– Engage the assistance of family members or an interpreter when English isn't the patient's primary language.
– Have them ask the patient to explain a saying in his native language.

Test the patient's judgment by asking him how he would respond to a hypothetical situation.
– What would he do if he was in a public building and the fire alarm sounded?
– Evaluate the appropriateness of his answer.

Throughout the interview, assess the patient's emotional status and note:
– mood
– emotional lability or stability
– appropriateness of his emotional responses.

Assess the patient's mood by asking how he feels about himself and his future.
– The symptoms of depression in elderly patients may be different from symptoms seen in younger patients.
– Elderly patients may exhibit decreased function or increased agitation instead of the usual sad affect of depressed people.

Constructional ability

- Assess the patient's ability to:
  - perform simple tasks
  - use various objects.

Assessing cranial nerve function

- Cranial nerves (CNs) transmit motor or sensory messages, or both, primarily between the brain and brain stem and between the head and neck.

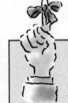

Memory jogger

Use the following mnemonic to help you remember which cranial nerves have sensory functions (S), motor functions (M), or both (B). The mnemonic begins with CN I and ends with CN XII:

I: Some	V: But	IX: Bad
II: Say	VI: My	X: Business
III: Marry	VII: Brother	XI: Marries
IV: Money	VIII: Says	XII: Money

Cranial nerve I

- Assess CN I, the olfactory nerve, first.
- Make sure the patient's nostrils are patent.
- Ask him to identify at least two common substances, such as coffee, cinnamon, or cloves.
- Avoid stringent odors, such as ammonia or peppermint, which stimulate the trigeminal nerve.

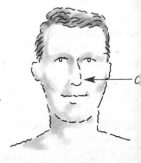

Cranial nerve II

CN II is the optic nerve.
To test the patient's visual acuity quickly and informally:
- Have the patient read a newspaper.
- Tell him to start with large headlines and then move to small print.

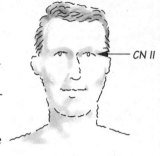

Test visual fields with a technique called *confrontation*.
- Stand 2′ (0.6 m) in front of the patient.
- Ask him to cover one eye.
- Close your eye on the side directly facing the patient's closed eye and bring your moving fingers into the patient's visual field from the periphery.
- Ask him to tell you when he sees the object.
- Test each quadrant of the patient's visual field, and compare his results with your own.

Examine the fundus of the optic nerve.
- Blurring of the optic disc may indicate increased intracranial pressure (ICP).

Cranial nerves III, IV, and VI

The oculomotor nerve (CN III), the trochlear nerve (CN IV), and the abducent nerve (CN VI) control eye movement.
- The oculomotor nerve controls most extraocular movement and is responsible for elevation of the eyelid and pupillary constriction.
- The trochlear nerve is responsible for down and in eye movement.
- The abducent nerve is responsible for lateral eye movement.

Visual field defects

Here are some examples of visual field defects. The black areas represent visual loss.

	Left	Right
A: Blindness in the right eye		
B: Bitemporal hemianopsia, or loss of one-half of the visual field		
C: Left homonymous hemianopsia		
D: Left homonymous hemianopsia in the superior quadrant		

- Assess these nerves together.
  - Ask the patient to follow your finger through the six cardinal positions of gaze: left superior, left lateral, left inferior, right superior, right lateral, and right inferior.
  - Pause slightly before moving from one position to the next; this helps to assess the patient for involuntary eye movement and the ability to hold his gaze in a that particular position.
  - Pupils should constrict when exposed to light, and the eye should accommodate to seeing objects at various distances.
- Oculomotor nerve abnormalities include:
  - ptosis (drooping of the upper lid)
  - pupil inequality.

Cranial nerve V

The trigeminal nerve (CN V) is both a sensory and a motor nerve. It supplies sensation to:
- corneas
- nasal and oral mucosa
- facial skin.

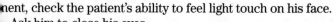

It supplies motor function for the jaw and all chewing muscles.

To assess the sensory component, check the patient's ability to feel light touch on his face.
- Ask him to close his eyes.
- Touch him with a wisp of cotton on his forehead, cheek, and jaw on each side.
- Test pain perception by touching the tip of a safety pin to the same three areas.
- Ask the patient to describe and compare both sensations.
- Alternate the touches between sharp and dull to test the patient's reliability in comparing sensations.
- Proper assessment of the nerve requires that the patient identify sharp stimuli.

To test the motor component:
- Ask the patient to clench his teeth.
- Palpate the temporal and masseter muscles.

Cranial nerve VII

The facial nerve (CN VII) has a sensory and motor component. The sensory component controls taste perception on the anterior part of the tongue.

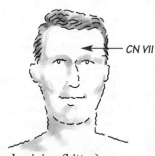

To assess taste:
- Place items with various tastes on the anterior portion of the patient's tongue, for example, sugar (sweet), salt, lemon juice (sour), and quinine (bitter).

– Ask the patient to identify the tastes.
– After each taste, have the patient clean his mouth by rinsing with a sip of water.
- The motor component of the facial nerve is responsible for the facial muscles.
- Assess the motor component by observing the patient's face for symmetry while he:
  – is at rest
  – smiles
  – frowns
  – raises his eyebrows.
- If a weakness caused by a stroke or other condition damages the cortex, the patient will be able to raise his eyebrows and wrinkle his forehead.
- If the weakness is due to an interruption of the facial nerve or other peripheral nerve involvement, the entire side of the face will be immobile.

Cranial nerve VIII

- The acoustic nerve (CN VIII) has two divisions.
  – The cochlear division controls hearing.
  – The vestibular division controls balance.

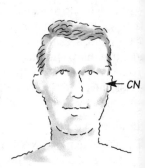

← CN

- To test the patient's hearing:
  – Ask him to cover one ear.
  – Stand on his opposite side.
  – Whisper a few words.
  – Ask him to repeat what you said.
  – Test the other ear the same way.
- To test the vestibular portion of this nerve:
  – Observe the patient for nystagmus and disturbed balance.
  – Note reports of dizziness or the room spinning.

Cranial nerves IX and X

The glossopharyngeal nerve (CN IX) is responsible for:
- swallowing
- salivation
- taste perception on the posterior one-third of the tongue.

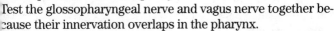

The vagus nerve (CN X):
- controls swallowing
- is responsible for voice quality.

Test the glossopharyngeal nerve and vagus nerve together because their innervation overlaps in the pharynx.
- Listen to the patient's voice.
- Check his gag reflex by asking the patient to open his mouth wide and say "ah." Then touch the tip of a tongue blade against his posterior pharynx.
- Watch for the symmetrical upward movement of the soft palate and uvula and for the midline position of the uvula.

Cranial nerve XI

The spinal accessory nerve (CN XI) is a motor nerve that controls:
- the sternocleidomastoid muscles
- the upper portion of the trapezius muscle.

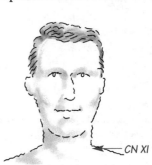

To assess this nerve, test the strength of both the muscles.
To test the sternocleidomastoid muscle:
- Place your palm against the patient's cheek.
- Ask him to turn his head against your resistance.
To test the trapezius muscle:
- Place your hands on the patient's shoulder.
- Ask him to shrug his shoulders against your resistance.

- Repeat each test on the other side, comparing muscle strength.

Cranial nerve XII

- The hypoglossal nerve (CN XII) controls tongue movement involved in swallowing and speech.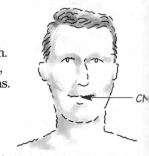
- Tongue should be at the midline, without tremors or fasciculations.
- Test tongue strength:
  – Ask the patient to push his tongue against his cheek as you apply resistance.
  – Observe the tongue for symmetry.

CN

Assessing sensory function

- Sensory system evaluation involves checking five areas of sensation:
  – pain
  – light touch
  – vibration
  – position
  – discrimination

Testing for pain sensation

- Have the patient close his eyes.
- Touch all the major dermatomes—first with the sharp end a safety pin and then with the dull end.
- Proceed in this order:
  – fingers
  – shoulders
  – toes
  – thighs
  – trunk.
- Ask him to tell you when he feels the sharp stimulus.
- If the patient has major deficits:

– Start in the area with the least sensation.
– Move toward the area with the most sensation to help you
determine the level of deficit.

Testing for the sense of light touch

Follow the same routine used to test for pain sensation but
use a wisp of cotton.
Lightly touch the patient's skin. Don't swab or sweep the cotton because you might miss an area of loss.
Patients with peripheral neuropathy might retain the sensation of light touch after pain sensation is lost.

Testing vibratory sense

Apply a tuning fork over
certain bony promi-
nences while the pa-
tient keeps his eyes
closed.
Start at the distal in-
terphalangeal joint of
the index finger and
move proximally.
Test only until the pa-
tient feels the vibra-
tion.
– Everything above
where the patient feels
the vibration is intact.
– If the vibratory sense
is intact, you won't
have to check position
sense because the
same pathway carries
both sensations.

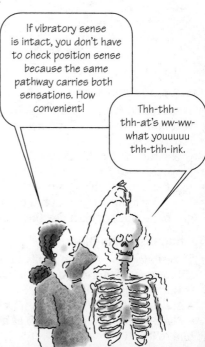

If vibratory sense
is intact, you don't have
to check position sense
because the same
pathway carries both
sensations. How
convenient!

Thh-thh-
thh-at's ww-ww-
what youuuuu
thh-thh-ink.

Evaluating vibratory sense

- Apply the base of a vibrating tuning fork to the interphalangeal joint of the patient's great toe, as shown at right.
- Ask him what he feels.
  - If he feels the sensation, he'll typically report a feeling of buzzing or vibration.
  - If he doesn't feel the sensation at the toe, try the medial malleolus.
  - Continue moving proximally until he feels the sensation.
- Note where he feels the sensation.
- Repeat the process on the other leg.

Testing position sense

- To be tested for position sense, the patient needs intact vestibular and cerebellar function.
- Have the patient close his eyes.
- Grasp the sides of his big toe.
- Move the toe up and down.
- Ask the patient what position the toe is in.
- To perform the same test on the patient's upper extremities, grasp the sides of his index finger and move it back and forth.

Testing discrimination

- To test *stereognosis*, the ability to discriminate the shape, size, weight, texture, and form of an object by touching and manipulating it:
  - Ask the patient to close his eyes and open his hand.
  - Place a common object, such as a key, in his hand and ask him to identify it.

– If he can't identify the object, test graphesthesia (the ability to recognize shapes, symbols or words when they're traced onto the skin).

To test graphesthesia:

– Tell the patient to keep his eyes closed and hold out his hand while you draw a large number on the palm.

– Ask him to identify the number.

To test point localization:

– Ask the patient to close his eyes.

– Touch one of his limbs.

– Ask him where you touched him.

Test two-point discrimination by touching the patient simultaneously in two contralateral areas.

– He should be able to identify both touches.

– Failure to perceive touch on one side is called *extinction*.

Assessing motor function

Muscle tone

Muscle tone represents muscular resistance to passive stretching

To test arm muscle tone:

– Move the patient's shoulder through passive range-of-motion (ROM) exercises.

– You should feel a slight resistance.

– Let the arm drop to the patient's side; it should fall easily.

To test leg muscle tone:

– Guide the hip through passive ROM exercises.

– Let the leg fall to the bed; the leg shouldn't fall into an externally rotated position.

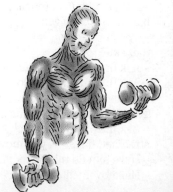

To assess motor function, you'll evaluate muscle tone and strength.

Muscle strength

- To perform a general examination of muscle strength, observe the patient's:
  - gait
  - motor activities.
- To evaluate muscle strength:
  - Ask the patient to move major muscles and muscle groups against resistance; for instance, to test shoulder girdle strength, have him extend his arms with his palms up and maintain this position for 30 seconds.
  - If he can't maintain this position, test further by pushing down on his outstretched arms.
  - If the patient lifts both arms equally, look for pronation of the hand and downward drift of the arm on the weaker side

Cerebellum

- Cerebellar testing is done because the cerebellum plays a role in smooth-muscle movements, such as tics, tremors, or fasciculations.
- Testing helps you evaluate the patient's coordination and general balance.
  - Can he sit and stand without support? If so, observe him as he walks across the room, turns, and walks back.
  - Note any imbalances or abnormalities.
  - A patient with cerebellar dysfunction will have a wide-based, unsteady gait.
  - Deviation to one side may indicate a cerebellar lesion on that side.
  - Ask the patient to walk heel to toe, and observe his balance
  - Ask the patient to follow your instructions to perform Romberg's test.
- Test the patient's extremity coordination.
  - Ask the patient to touch his nose and then touch your outstretched finger as you move it.
  - Have him do this faster and faster.
  - His movements should be accurate and smooth.

Romberg's test

Observe the patient's balance as he stands with his eyes open, feet together, and arms at his sides.

Ask him to close his eyes.

Hold your arms out on either side of him to protect him if he sways.

If he falls to one side, the result of the Romberg's test is positive.

Assess rapid alternating movements.
- Ask the patient to touch the thumb of his right hand to his right index finger and then to each of his remaining fingers.
- The patient's movements should be accurate and smooth.
- Ask him to sit with his palms on his thighs.
- Tell him to turn his palms up and down, gradually increasing his speed.
- Next, ask the patient to lie down in a supine position.
- Stand at the foot of the table or bed and hold your palms near the soles of his feet.
- Ask him to alternately tap the sole of his right foot and the sole of his left foot against your palms.
- Tell him to increase his speed.

Assessing reflexes

Deep tendon reflexes

Make sure the patient is relaxed and the joint is flexed appropriately.

Distract the patient by asking him to focus on a point across the room.

Always test by moving from head to toe and comparing side to side.

Grade deep tendon reflexes using this scale: 0 indicates absent impulses; +1 indicates diminished impulses; +2 indi-

Help desk

5¢

Assessing deep tendon reflexes

Biceps reflex
• Position the patient's arm with his elbow flexed at a 45-degree angle and his arm relaxed.
• Place your thumb or index finger over the biceps tendon and your remaining fingers loosely over the triceps muscle.
• Strike your finger with the pointed end of the reflex hammer; watch and feel for the contraction of the biceps muscle and flexion of the forearm.

Triceps reflex
• Have the patient adduct his arm and place his forearm across his chest.
• Strike the triceps tendon about 2″ (5 cm) above the olecranon process on the extensor surface of the upper arm.
• Watch for contraction of the triceps muscle and extension of the forearm.

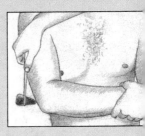

cates normal impulses; +3 indicates increased impulses (m be normal); +4 indicates hyperactive impulses.

Superficial reflexes

• To test superficial reflexes, stimulate the skin or mucous membranes.
• Because these are cutaneous reflexes, the more you try to elicit them in succession, the less response you'll get.
• Observe the patient carefully the first time you stimulate a cation.

Assessing deep tendon reflexes *(continued)*

Brachioradialis reflex
Ask the patient to rest the ulnar surface of his hand on his abdomen or lap with the elbow partially flexed.
Strike the radius.
Watch for supination of the hand and flexion of the forearm at the elbow.

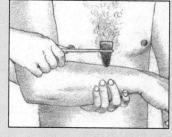

Patellar reflex
Have the patient sit with his legs dangling freely.
If he can't sit up, flex his knee at a 45-degree angle and place your nondominant hand behind the knee for support.
Strike the patellar tendon just below the patella.
Look for contraction of the quadriceps muscle in the thigh with extension of the leg.

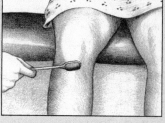

Achilles reflex
Have the patient flex his foot.
Support the plantar surface.
Strike the Achilles tendon.
Watch for the plantar flexion of the foot at the ankle.

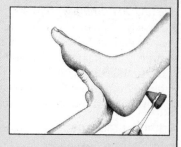

Testing superficial reflexes in the feet
- Slowly stroke the lateral side of the patient's sole from the heel to the great toe using an applicator stick, tongue blade or key.
- Normal response in an adult is plantar flexion of the toes.
- Upward movement of the great toe and fanning of the little toes (Babinski's reflex) is abnormal.

Babinski's reflex in infants

The Babinski reflex can be elicited in some normal infants — sometimes until age 2 years. However, the plantar flexion of the toes is seen in more than 90% of normal infants.

Testing the cremasteric reflex in men
- Use an applicator stick to stimulate the inner thigh.
- The cremaster muscle should contract and the testicle show elevate on the side of the stimulus.

Testing abdominal reflexes
- Have the patient lie in the supine position with his arms at sides and his knees slightly flexed.
- Briskly stroke both sides of the abdomen above and below the umbilicus.
- Move from the periphery toward the midline.
- Movement of the umbilicus toward the stimulus is normal.

Primitive reflexes
- Primitive reflexes are:
  – abnormal in an adult
  – normal in an infant, whose central nervous system is imm ture.

They disappear as the nervous system matures.
Primitive reflexes include:
- grasp
- snout
- sucking
- glabella.

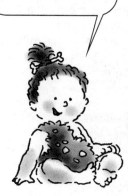

Primitive reflexes are normal for someone my age, but they're abnormal in an adult.

Assessing for the grasp reflex

Apply gentle pressure to the patient's palm with your fingers.
If he grasps your fingers between his index finger and thumb, suspect cortical or premotor cortex damage.

Assessing for the snout reflex

Lightly tap the patient's upper lip.
Pursing of the lip is a positive snout reflex that indicates frontal lobe damage.

Assessing for the sucking reflex

Observe the patient while you're feeding him.
If you see a sucking motion, the sucking reflex is positive.
If the patient has an oral airway or endotracheal tube in place and you see a sucking motion, the sucking reflex is positive.
A positive sucking reflex indicates cortical damage.
This reflex is commonly seen in patients with advanced dementia.

Assessing for the glabella response

Repeatedly tap the bridge of the patient's nose.
Persistent blinking is an abnormal response and indicates diffuse cortical dysfunction.

Abnormal findings

Altered level of consciousness

- May result from any one of several factors that can affect the cerebral hemisphere of the brain stem, including:
  - toxic encephalopathy
  - hemorrhage
  - extensive, generalized cortical atrophy
  - compression of brain-stem structures from tumor, swelling, or hemorrhage
  - sedatives
  - opioids
- Is the most sensitive indicator of neurologic dysfunction
- May be a valuable adjunct to other findings
- Is assessed by using a stimulus that's strong enough to get a true picture of the patient's baseline

Cranial nerve impairment

Olfactory impairment

- Involves an inability to detect odors with both nostrils
- Occurs with dysfunction in CN I
- Can result from any condition that affects the olfactory tract such as:
  - tumor
  - hemorrhage
  - facial bone fracture that crosses the cribriform plate (the portion of the ethmoid bone that separates the roof of the nose from the cranial cavity)

Visual impairment

Visual field defects

- May result from tumors or infarcts of the optic nerve head, optic chiasm, or optic tracts

(Text continues on page 306)

Between the lines

Evaluating neurologic findings

Sign or symptom and findings	Probable cause
Aphasia	
Wernicke's, Broca's, or global aphasia Decreased LOC Right-sided hemiparesis Homonymous hemianopsia Paresthesia and loss of sensation	Stroke
Any type of aphasia occurring suddenly (may be transient or permanent) Blurred or double vision Headache Cerebrospinal otorrhea and rhinorrhea Disorientation Behavioral changes Signs of increased ICP	Head trauma
Any type of aphasia occurring suddenly and resolving within 24 hours Transient hemiparesis Hemianopsia Paresthesia Dizziness and confusion	Transient ischemic attack
Decreased LOC	
Slowly decreasing LOC, from lethargy to coma Apathy and behavior changes Memory loss Decreased attention span Morning headache Sensorimotor disturbances	Brain tumor

(continued)

Evaluating neurologic findings (continued)

Sign or symptom and findings	Probable caus
Decreased LOC (continued)	
• Slowly decreasing LOC, from lethargy possibly to coma • Malaise • Tachycardia • Tachypnea • Orthostatic hypotension • Hot, flushed, and diaphoretic skin	Heatstroke
• Lethargy progressing to coma • Confusion, anxiety, and restlessness • Hypotension • Tachycardia • Weak pulse with narrowing pulse pressure • Dyspnea • Oliguria • Cool, clammy skin	Shock
Tremors • Tremors in fingers, which progress to the feet, eyelids, jaws, lips, and tongue • Characteristic pill-rolling tremor • Lead-pipe rigidity • Bradykinesia • Propulsive gait with forward-leaning posture • Masklike face • Drooling	Parkinson's disease

valuating neurologic findings (continued)

gn or symptom and findings	Probable cause
emors (continued)	
Intention tremor that comes and goes Visual and sensory impairments Muscle weakness, paralysis, or spasticity Hyperreflexia Ataxic gait Dysphagia Dysarthria	Multiple sclerosis
Intention tremor Ataxia Nystagmus Muscle weakness and atrophy Hypoactive or absent deep tendon reflexes	Cerebellar tumor
praxia	
Gradual and irreversible apraxia Amnesia Anomia Decreased attention span Apathy Aphasia	Alzheimer's disease
Progressive apraxia Decreased mental activity Headache Dizziness Seizures Pupillary changes	Brain tumor

(continued)

Evaluating neurologic findings *(continued)*	
Sign or symptom and findings	**Probable caus**
Apraxia *(continued)* • Sudden onset of apraxia • Headache • Confusion • Aphasia • Agnosia • Stupor or coma • Hemiplegia • Visual field defects	Stroke

Pupillary changes

- May indicate neurologic dysfunction
- Include:
  – changes in pupillary response to light, which can indicate damage to the optic nerve and oculomotor nerve
  – dilated pupil ipsilateral to a mass or lesion (such as those caused by cancer, benign tumor growth, or hematomas), which indicates increased ICP; without treatment, this condition can lead to both pupils being fixed and dilated
  – unequal pupils, or *anisocoria*, in which pupil size doesn't change with the amount of illumination (normal in about 20 of people)

Eye muscle impairment

- Can result from cranial nerve damage
- Involves conditions such as:
  – nystagmus (eyes drift slowly in one direction and then jer back to the other) resulting from damage to the peripheral labyrinth, brain stem, or cerebellum

Detecting increased ICP

The earlier you recognize the signs of increased ICP, the quicker you can intervene. The sooner the intervention, the better chance the patient has of recovery. By the time late signs appear, interventions may not help the patient.

	Early signs	Late signs
Level of consciousness	• Requires increased stimulation • A subtle loss of orientation • Restlessness and anxiety • Suddenly quiet	• Can't be aroused
Pupils	• Pupil changes on the side of the lesion • One pupil constricts but then dilates (unilateral hippus) • A sluggish reaction in both pupils • Unequal pupils	• Pupils fixed and dilated or "blown"
Motor response	• Sudden weakness • Motor changes on the side opposite the lesion • A positive pronator drift; with palms up, one hand pronates	• Profound weakness
Vital signs	• Intermittent increases in blood pressure	• Increased systolic pressure, profound bradycardia, and abnormal respirations (Cushing's triad)

Types of pupillary changes

Pupillary change	Possible causes
Unilateral, dilated (4 mm), fixed, and nonreactive 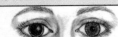	• Uncal herniation with oculomotor nerve damage • Brain stem compression • An increase in ICP • Tentorial herniation • Head trauma with subdural or epidural hematoma • Normal in some people
Bilateral, dilated (4 mm), fixed, and nonreactive 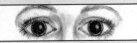	• Severe midbrain damage • Cardiopulmonary arrest (hypoxia) • Anticholinergic poisoning
Bilateral, midsize (2 mm), fixed, and nonreactive 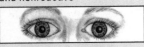	• Midbrain involvement caused by edema, hemorrhage, infarctions, lacerations, and contusions
Bilateral, pinpoint (less than 1 mm), and usually nonreactive 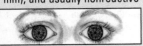	• Lesions of pons, which usually occur after a hemorrhage
Unilateral, small (1.5 mm), and nonreactive 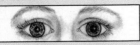	• Disruption of the sympathetic nerv supply to the head caused by a spin cord lesion above the first thoracic vertebra

- problems with the motor nuclei of the oculomotor, trochlear, and abducent nerves caused by increased ICP and intracranial lesions
- ptosis (drooping of the eyelid) resulting from a defect in the oculomotor nerve
- weakness or paralysis of the eye muscles

Facial nerve impairment

May involve the trigeminal nerve if the patient responds inadequately to sensory stimulation of the skin or eye
Includes trigeminal neuralgia, which causes severe piercing or stabbing pain over one or more of the facial dermatomes

Sensorial hearing loss

Can result from:
- lesions of the cochlear branch of the acoustic nerve
- lesions in any part of the nerve's pathway
to the brain stem
May involve:
- total loss of hearing in the affected ear
- trouble hearing high-pitched sounds

Aphasia

Speech disorder
Caused by injury to the cerebral cortex

Expressive aphasia

Also called *Broca's aphasia*
Involves impaired fluency and difficulty finding words
Affects the frontal lobe, the anterior speech area

Receptive aphasia

Also called *Wernicke's aphasia*
Involves the inability to understand written words or speech
and the use of made-up words

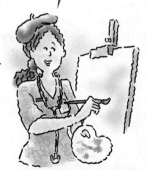

Is your patient having trouble expressing himself? He may have expressive aphasia.

- Caused by impairment in the posterior speech cortex, which involves the temporal and parietal lobes

Global aphasia
- Involves lack of both expressive and receptive language
- Results from impairment of both speech areas

Constructional impairment

Apraxia
- Inability to perform purposeful movements and make proper use of objects
- Commonly associated with parietal lobe dysfunction
- Can be one of four types:
  - *constructional apraxia*—inability to copy a design such as the face of a clock
  - *dressing apraxia*—inability to understand the meaning of various articles of clothing or the sequence of actions required to get dressed
  - *ideational apraxia*—awareness of actions that should be done but inability to perform them
  - *ideomotor apraxia*—inability to understand the effect of motor activity; ability to perform simple activities but without awareness of performing them; inability to perform actions on command

Agnosia
- Inability to identify common objects
- May indicate a lesion in the sensory cortex
- Can be one of three types:
  - *visual*—inability to identify common objects without touching
  - *auditory*—inability to identify common sounds
  - *body image*—inability to identify body parts by sight or touch; inability to localize a stimulus; denial of existence of one-half of the body

Vertigo

The illusion of movement
Can result from a disturbance of the vestibular centers
If caused by a peripheral lesion:
– occurs along with nystagmus 10 to 20 seconds after the patient changes position
– gradually lessens with the repetition of the position change
If of central origin:
– has no latent period
– has no diminishing of symptoms with repetition

Dysphagia

Difficulty swallowing
Commonly occurs after stroke
Can result from a mass lesion affecting CN IX and CN X

Abnormal muscle movements

Tics

Sudden, uncontrolled movements of the face, shoulders, and extremities
Caused by abnormal neural stimuli
May manifest as normal movements that appear repetitively and inappropriately, such as:
– blinking
– shoulder shrugging
– facial twitching

Tremors

Involuntary, repetitive movements
Usually seen in:
– fingers
– wrist
– eyelids
– tongue
– legs

- Can occur:
  – when the affected body part is at rest (as in the characteristic pill-rolling resting tremor of Parkinson's disease)
  – with voluntary movement (as in the intention tremor a patient with cerebellar disease has when reaching for an object)

Lower motor neuron dysfunction can lead to fasciculations.

Fasciculations

- Slight twitchings of muscle fibers that can be seen under the skin
- Most commonly associated with lower motor neuron dysfunction

Abnormal gaits

- May result from disorders of the:
  – cerebellum
  – posterior columns
  – corticospinal tract
  – basal ganglia
  – lower motor neurons

Spastic gait

- Sometimes referred to as *paretic* or *weak gait*
- Stiff, foot-dragging walk
- Caused by unilateral leg muscle hypertonicity
- Occurs because leg doesn't swing normally at the hip or knee, so the foot tends to drag or shuffle, scraping the toes on the ground
- Indicates focal damage to the corticospinal tract
- Usually permanent

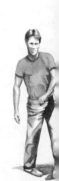

cissors gait

Results from bilateral spastic paresis
Affects both legs
Has little or no effect on the arms
Appears as legs flexing slightly at the hips and
knees, so patient looks as if he's crouching
Causes a scissorslike movement with each
step because the thighs adduct and the knees
hit or cross

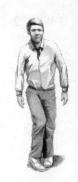

ropulsive gait

Characterized by a stooped, rigid posture,
including:
– head and neck that are bent forward
– flexed, stiffened arms that are held away
from the body
– extended fingers
– stiffly bent knees and hips
Cardinal sign of advanced Parkinson's disease

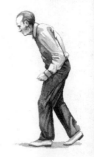

teppage gait

Typically results from footdrop, which causes the foot to hang with the toes pointing
down so they scrape the ground during am-
bulation
Involves:
– exaggerated flexion of hip and knee to lift
the advancing leg off the ground
– outward rotation of the hip
Produces an audible slap because foot is
thrown forward and the toes hit the ground
first

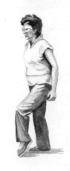

Waddling gait

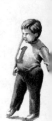

- Distinctive ducklike walk
- Can signal:
  – muscular dystrophy
  – spinal muscle atrophy
  – developmental dysplasia of the hip
- May be present when the child begins to walk
- May appear only later in life
- Results from deterioration of the pelvic girdle muscles

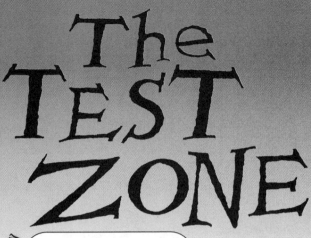

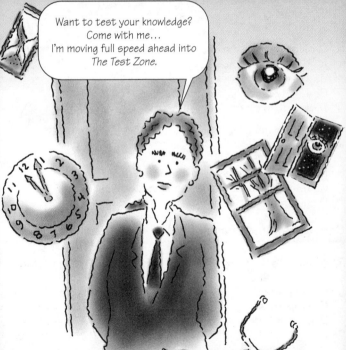

Want to test your knowledge?
Come with me...
I'm moving full speed ahead into
The Test Zone.

Chapter 1: Health history

1. Which form of nonverbal communication might a patient from
Arabic-speaking country find disrespectful?
  A. Nodding your head
  B. Making eye contact
  C. Touching him
  D. Facing him while standing 3′ to 4′ (0.9 to 1.2 m) away

2. Which communication technique involves the nurse repeating
what the patient said?
  A. Facilitation
  B. Clarification
  C. Confirmation
  D. Reflection

3. Which element of a health history is considered biographic da
  A. Chief complaint
  B. Past medical problems
  C. Emergency contact person
  D. Family history

4. A psychosocial history helps determine how the patient feels
about:
  A. his illness.
  B. his ability to pay for medical care.
  C. himself and his relationship with others.
  D. his treatment plan.

Chapter 2: Fundamentals of physical assessment

5. Which physical assessment technique should you perform firs
  A. Palpation
  B. Auscultation
  C. Inspection
  D. Percussion

The pulse deficit is the difference between:
A. systolic blood pressure and radial pulse rate.
B. systolic and diastolic blood pressure.
C. systolic blood pressure and atrial pulse rate.
D. apical and radial pulse rates.

Which intervention should be performed before auscultating rt sounds of a patient who has hair on his chest?
A. Clip the hair with scissors.
B. Shave the hair with a razor.
C. Wet the hair lightly.
D. No intervention is necessary.

Which percussion sound is described as a drumlike sound that's rd over enclosed air?
A. Tympany
B. Resonance
C. Hyperresonance
D. Dullness

apter 3: Nutritional assessment

What's a primary energy source for the body?
A. Vitamins
B. Protein
C. Fat
D. Minerals

You calculate a BMI of 26 in your patient admitted with hyper-sion. Based on the BMI definitions, your patient would be classi-as:
A. overweight.
B. obese.
C. underweight.
D. normal weight.

11. Which statement about the serum transferrin level is true?
  A. It helps assess the blood's oxygen-carrying capacity.
  B. It determines the difference between nitrogen intake and e
     cretion.
  C. It helps determine the patient's risk of coronary artery dis-
     ease.
  D. It reflects the patient's protein status more accurately than
     serum albumin level.

12. Which finding is a primary sign of an endocrine disorder?
  A. Anorexia
  B. Excessive weight gain
  C. Muscle wasting
  D. Excessive weight loss

Chapter 4: Mental health assessment

13. Which mental status test assesses and stages primary degene
tive dementia?
  A. Cognitive Capacity Screening Examination
  B. Global Deterioration Scale
  C. Cognitive Assessment Scale
  D. Mini-Mental Status Examination

14. Your patient's speech vacillates from one subject another. Wh
term would you use to document this abnormal thought process'
  A. Echolalia
  B. Flight of ideas
  C. Confabulation
  D. Derailment

15. A patient tells you that he has recurrent, uncontrollable
thoughts about washing his hands. Which term is used to describ
this abnormal thought content?
  A. Obsession
  B. Compulsion
  C. Phobia
  D. Delusion

As you attempt to begin your admission interview, the patient ins to yell at you, "Why did you treat me so badly?" Which cop- mechanism is the patient using?

A. Identification
B. Reaction formation
C. Projection
D. Displacement

apter 5: Skin, hair, and nails

Which skin condition may be exacerbated by increased skin perature, poor skin turgor, and stress?

A. Urticaria
B. Vesicular rash
C. Pruritus
D. Ecchymoses

The mother of a neonate asks you when her baby will lose the hair that's covering his body. You tell her that lanugo (fine, vny growth of hair) is typically shed:

A. within 3 days of birth.
B. within 1 week of birth.
C. within 2 weeks of birth.
D. within 3 weeks of birth.

Rough, dry skin is associated with which disorder?

A. Hypothyroidism
B. Diabetes mellitus
C. Hyperkalemia
D. Heart failure

The nurse is assessing a patient admitted with subacute bacteri- ndocarditis. She notes red, pinpoint lesions on the patient's ik. Which term should the nurse use to document this finding?

A. Telangiectases
B. Petechiae
C. Ecchymoses
D. Hematoma

Chapter 6: Eyes

21. Which disorder is a cause of vision loss?
A. Strabismus
B. Diabetic retinopathy
C. Amblyopia
D. Refractory errors

22. A patient complains to the nurse about seeing yellow halos around bright lights. The nurse should suspect:
A. corneal abrasion.
B. foreign body in the eye.
C. digoxin overdose.
D. chemical agent exposure.

23. Which test helps evaluate the oculomotor, trigeminal, and abdcent nerves as well as the extraocular muscles?
A. Cover-uncover test
B. Corneal light reflex
C. Confrontation test
D. Cardinal positions of gaze

24. The nurse is assessing a patient's eyes and notes drooping of upper eyelid. What term should the nurse use to document her findi
A. Diplopia
B. Ptosis
C. Strabismus
D. Hyperopia

Chapter 7: Ears, nose, and throat

25. Which lobe of the cerebral cortex interprets sound?
A. Temporal lobe
B. Occipital lobe
C. Frontal lobe
D. Parietal lobe

Which ear inspection finding commonly accompanies congenital
rders?

A. Both ears have an angle of attachment of 10 degrees.

B. Auricles protrude from the head.

C. Ears are low-set.

D. Face and ears are different colors.

A patient comes to the clinic complaining of difficulty swallow-
The nurse should document this assessment finding as:

A. epistaxis.

B. dysphagia.

C. dysphasia.

D. pharyngitis.

The nurse is assessing the mouth and throat of a dark-skinned
ent when she notes flecked pigmentation on the lips. What does
finding suggest?

A. It's a normal finding in dark-skinned patients.

B. The patient has a coagulation disorder.

C. The patient has a renal disorder.

D. The patient is dehydrated.

apter 8: Respiratory system

Which question should the nurse include when asking the
ent about orthopnea?

A. "Do you cough up blood?"

B. "Does it move to another area?"

C. "Is it sharp, stabbing, burning, or aching?"

D. "How many pillows do you use?"

Which muscle is considered a primary muscle used in respira-
?

A. Scalene

B. Diaphragm

C. Trapezius

D. Sternocleidomastoid

31. Which assessment finding is commonly described as a feeling puffed-rice cereal crackling under the skin?
    A. Crepitus
    B. Tactile fremitus
    C. Resonance
    D. Egophony

32. A 23-year-old patient is admitted with head trauma. While assessing the patient, the nurse notes rapid, deep breaths that alt nate with abrupt periods of apnea. What term should the nurse u to document her findings?
    A. Cheyne-Stokes respirations
    B. Biot's respirations
    C. Kussmaul's respirations
    D. Hyperpnea

Chapter 9: Cardiovascular system

33. Blood from the superior vena cava, inferior vena cava, and co nary sinus empties into which chamber of the heart?
    A. Left atrium
    B. Right atrium
    C. Left ventricle
    D. Right ventricle

34. How should the patient be positioned before beginning a car vascular assessment?
    A. Supine
    B. Left lateral
    C. Prone
    D. Supine with the head of the bed elevated 30 to 45 degrees

35. Where should the nurse position the stethoscope to best ausc tate the first heart sound (S_1)?
    A. Over the tricuspid valve
    B. Over the mitral valve
    C. Over the apex of the heart
    D. Over the aortic valve

While performing a cardiovascular assessment, the nurse notes
palpable vibration over the mitral valve. What term should the
nurse use to document this finding?

A. Thrill
B. Heave
C. Murmur
D. Friction rub

apter 10: Breasts and axillae

Which substance has been linked to fibrocystic breast disease?

A. Aspartame
B. Nicotine
C. Caffeine
D. Estrogen

The nurse asks the patient to lie in a supine position before pal-
ng the breast. What else should the nurse do before performing
pation?

A. Elevate the head of the bed or examination table to 45 de-
   grees.
B. Place a small pillow under the patient's shoulder on the side
   where she's examining the breast.
C. Have the patient place her hands on her hips.
D. Put on gloves.

Which assessment finding is a late sign of breast cancer?

A. Nipple retraction
B. Breast pain
C. Visible veins
D. Peau d'orange

Which action should the nurse take after palpating the breast?

A. Put on gloves.
B. Squeeze the nipple to check for discharge.
C. Have the patient put her hand behind her head.
D. Inspect the breasts as the patient holds her arms over her
   head.

Chapter 11: Gastrointestinal system

41. Where in the GI system are carbohydrates, fats, and proteins broken down?
  A. Large intestine
  B. Liver
  C. Small intestine
  D. Stomach

42. If the patient's chief complaint is diarrhea, the nurse should a about:
  A. laxative use.
  B. excessive passing of gas.
  C. allergies to medications.
  D. recent travel abroad.

43. Visible, rippling waves in the abdomen may suggest:
  A. bowel obstruction.
  B. aortic insufficiency.
  C. aortic aneurysm.
  D. normal peristalsis.

44. The nurse is caring for a patient who underwent liver transplantation 6 weeks ago. Which assessment technique should the nurse avoid when performing an abdominal assessment on this patient?
  A. Auscultation
  B. Palpation
  C. Inspection
  D. Percussion

Chapter 12: Female genitourinary system

45. Which assessment finding may signal renal dysfunction?
  A. Unexplained weight gain
  B. Frequent urination at night
  C. Pain during urination
  D. Urinary incontinence

Where does fertilization of the ova by the sperm usually take ᴄe?

A. Vagina
B. Fallopian tubes
C. Ovaries
D. Cervix

A patient comes to the clinic complaining of abnormally frent urination. The nurse should use which term when reporting complaint to the doctor?

A. Urinary frequency
B. Nocturia
C. Dysuria
D. Urinary urgency

Which type of lesion may occur as genital warts progress?

A. Red, painless, eroding lesion with a raised indurated border
B. Small erythematous vesicular lesions
C. Multiple swellings with a cauliflower appearance
D. Multiple shallow vesicular lesions

apter 13: Male genitourinary system

Which assessment finding indicates possible decreased renal ᴄtion?

A. Keratinization
B. Nevi
C. Paleness
D. Purpura

A patient comes to the clinic complaining of a profuse, yellow ᴄharge from his penis. This finding is common with:

A. testicular tumor.
B. paraphimosis.
C. chlamydial infection.
D. gonococcal urethritis.

51. Which statement best describes a hydrocele?
   A. The urethral meatus is located on the top of the penis.
   B. Fluid has collected in the testicle.
   C. The prepuce is so tight that it gets caught behind the glans when retracted.
   D. The urethral meatus is located on the underside of the peni:

52. Which condition is a urologic emergency?
   A. Priapism
   B. Paraphimosis
   C. Hypospadias
   D. Epispadias

Chapter 14: Musculoskeletal system

53. What's the only special equipment needed to accurately asses: the musculoskeletal system?
   A. Penlight
   B. Stethoscope
   C. Tape measure
   D. Scale

54. The length of the spine from neck to waist usually increases by at least how many inches when the patient bends forward?
   A. 6″
   B. 4″
   C. 3″
   D. 2″

55. Which of the following findings occurs to some degree with aging?
   A. Foot drop
   B. Muscle spasms
   C. Crepitus
   D. Muscle atrophy

Which type of medication can cause muscle cramping?
A. Potassium-depleting diuretics
B. Angiotensin-converting enzyme inhibitors
C. Corticosteroids
D. Antihistamines

apter 15: Neurologic system

The brain stem is responsible for regulating which body func-
?
A. Ability to stand
B. Breathing
C. Water balance
D. Pituitary hormone production

The nurse is assessing a 70-year-old patient admitted with a sub-
chnoid hemorrhage. What's the most sensitive indicator of neuro-
c status change?
A. Pupillary response
B. Blood pressure
C. LOC
D. Cognitive function

Which cranial nerve is responsible for hearing and equilibrium?
A. V
B. VI
C. VII
D. VIII

The nurse notes a positive glabella response. This response indi-
s damage to which brain structure?
A. Cerebellum
B. Frontal lobe
C. Temporal lobe
D. Cortex

Answers

Chapter 1: Health history

1. B. Patients from certain cultural backgrounds, including those o Arabic-speaking countries, may consider eye contact disrespectful.

2. D. Reflection involves repeating what the patient just said, typic in the form of a question. This technique helps you to obtain more sp cific information about the patient.

3. C. The name and phone number of a person to contact in case o an emergency are considered biographic data.

4. C. A psychosocial history helps determine how the patient feels about himself, his place in society, and his relationship with others.

Chapter 2: Fundamentals of physical assessment

5. C. The assessment of each body system begins with inspection.

6. D. The pulse deficit is the difference between the apical and rad pulse rates. It provides an indirect evaluation of the ability of each h contraction to eject enough blood into the peripheral circulation.

7. C. Before auscultating heart sounds of a patient who has hair or his chest, wet the hair lightly to prevent interference.

8. A. Tympany is a drumlike sound heard over enclosed air. This sound signifies air in the bowel.

Chapter 3: Nutritional assessment

9. C. Carbohydrates and fat are the primary sources of energy for body; protein is a secondary source.

10. A. BMI between 25 and 29.9 is defined as overweight.

11. D. The serum transferrin level reflects the patient's protein statu more accurately than the serum albumin level.

12. B. Excessive weight gain is a primary sign of an endocrine disor

Chapter 4: Mental health assessment

13. B. The Global Deterioration Scale assesses and stages primary degenerative dementia based on orientation, memory, and neurologi function.

D. You should document your finding as derailment, an abnormal
ght process in which speech vacillates from one subject to another
lly unrelated subject.

A. An obsession is characterized by recurrent, uncontrollable
ghts, images, or impulses that the patient considers unaccept-
.

C. The patient is using the projection coping mechanism. He's dis-
ng negative feelings onto another person.

pter 5: Skin, hair, and nails

C. Pruritus may be exacerbated by increased skin temperature,
skin turgor, local vasodilation, dermatoses, and stress.

C. Most lanugo is shed within 2 weeks of birth.

A. Rough, dry skin is common with hypothyroidism.

B. The nurse should document her finding of red, pinpoint lesions
techiae.

pter 6: Eyes

B. Disorders that cause vision loss include diabetic retinopathy,
coma, cataracts, macular degeneration, opportunistic infections
ciated with human immunodeficiency infection, toxoplasmosis, and
negalovirus retinitis.

C. The nurse should suspect digoxin overdose in the patient who
plains of seeing yellow halos around bright lights.

D. The cardinal positions of gaze help evaluate the oculomotor,
minal, and abducent nerves as well as the extraocular muscles.

B. The nurse should document her finding as ptosis — drooping of
pper eyelid.

pter 7: Ears, nose, and throat

A. The cochlear branch of the acoustic nerve transmits the vibra-
to the temporal lobe of the cerebral cortex, where the brain inter-
the sound.

C. Low-set ears commonly accompany congenital disorders such as
y problems.

27. B. The nurse should document difficulty swallowing as dysphag

28. A. A bluish hue or flecked pigmentation on the lips is a normal 1 ing in dark-skinned individuals.

Chapter 8: Respiratory system

29. D. The nurse should ask the patient with orthopnea (shortness breath when lying down) how many pillows he uses.

30. B. The diaphragm is considered a primary muscle used in respi tion. The scalene, trapezius, and sternocleidomastoid muscles are a accessory muscles of respiration.

31. A. Crepitus, which indicates subcutaneous air in the chest, is fr quently described as a feeling of puffed-rice cereal crackling under t skin.

32. B. The nurse should document her findings as Biot's respiratior which are rapid, deep breaths that alternate with abrupt periods of apnea. This finding is a sign of severe central nervous system damaç

Chapter 9: Cardiovascular system

33. B. Blood from the superior vena cava, inferior vena cava, and t coronary sinus empties into the right atrium of the heart.

34. D. Have the patient lie in a supine position with the head of the or examination table elevated 30 to 45 degrees.

35. C. The S_1 heart sound is best heard over the apex of the heart.

36. A. The nurse should document her finding as a thrill, a palpable vibration that usually suggests a valvular dysfunction.

Chapter 10: Breasts and axillae

37. C. Caffeine has been linked to fibrocystic breast disease.

38. B. The nurse should place a small pillow under the shoulder on side where she's examining the breast.

39. D. Peau d'orange — edematous thickening and pitting of breast tissue — is a late sign of breast cancer.

40. A. The nurse should put on gloves and then palpate the areola a nipple. After doing so she should gently squeeze the nipple between thumb and index finger to check for discharge.

pter 11: Gastrointestinal system

C. Carbohydrates, fats, and proteins are broken down in the small
stine.

D. If the patient's chief complaint is diarrhea, the nurse should ask
ut recent travel abroad. Diarrhea can result from ingesting contami-
d food or water.

A. Visible, rippling waves may indicate bowel obstruction.

D. The nurse should avoid percussing the abdomen of a patient
a transplanted abdominal organ. Doing so can precipitate organ
ction.

pter 12: Female genitourinary system

A. Sudden, unexplained weight gain may suggest fluid retention, a
of renal dysfunction.

B. Fertilization usually occurs in the fallopian tubes.

A. The nurse should report this complaint as urinary frequency.

C. As genital warts progress, the patient may develop multiple
lings that have a cauliflower-like appearance.

pter 13: Male genitourinary system

C. Pale skin caused by a low hemoglobin level may indicate
eased renal function.

D. Profuse, yellow discharge from the penis suggests gonococcal
ritis.

B. A hydrocele is a collection of fluid in the testicle.

A. Priapism, a persistent, painful erection that's unrelated to sexual
ation, is considered a urologic emergency.

pter 14: Musculoskeletal system

C. The only special equipment necessary to perform a musculo-
tal assessment is a tape measure.

D. The length of the spine from neck to waist usually increases by
st 2″ when the patient bends forward; if it doesn't the patient's
lity may be impaired.

55. D. Some muscle atrophy is normal with aging.
56. A. Potassium-depleting diuretics can cause muscle cramping.

Chapter 15: Neurologic system

57. B. The brain stem regulates automatic body functions including heart rate, swallowing, breathing, and coughing.
58. C. A change in LOC is the earliest and most sensitive indicator t neurologic status has changed. The nurse should closely assess for s tle changes in the patient's LOC.
59. D. The acoustic nerve (cranial nerve VIII) is responsible for hea and equilibrium.
60. D. A positive glabella response indicates diffuse cortical dysfun tion, indicating damage to the cortex.

Scoring

☆☆☆ If you answered 55 to 60 questions correctly, great job!
You're in a dimension all by yourself.

☆☆ If you answered 45 to 54 questions correctly, way to go!
You're really in the zone.

☆ If you answered fewer than 45 questions correctly, revie
the chapters and try again! It won't be long until y
see the light.

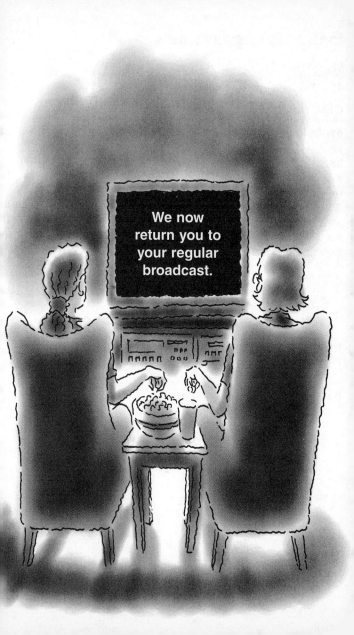

Selected references

Alcenius, M. "Successfully Meet Pain Assessment Standards," *Nursing Management* 35(3):12, March 2004.

Anatomy & Physiology Made Incredibly Easy, 2nd ed. Philadelphia: Lippincott Williams & Wilkins, 2005.

Andrews, M.M., and Boyle, J.S. *Transcultural Concepts in Nursing Care*, 4th ed. Philadelphia: Lippincott Williams & Wilkins, 2003.

Assessment: A 2-in-1 Reference for Nurses. Philadelphia: Lippincott Williams & Wilkins, 2004.

Bickley, L.S. *Bates' Guide to Physical Examination and History Taking*, 8th ed. Philadelphia: Lippincott Williams & Wilkins, 2005.

Bourbonnais, F.F., et al. "Introduction of a Pain and Symptom Assessment Tool in the Clinical Setting — Lessons Learned," *Journal of Nursing Management* 12(3):194-200, May 2004.

Coviello, J.S. "Cardiac Assessment 101: A New Look at the Guidelines for Cardiac Homecare Patients," *Home Healthcare Nurse* 22(2):116-23, February 2004.

Doughty, D.B. "Wound Assessment: Tips and Technique *Home Healthcare Nurse* 22(3):192-95, March 2004.

Giger, J.N., and Davidhizar, R.F *Transcultural Nursing: Assessment and Intervention*, 4th ed. St. Louis Mosby–Year Book, Inc., 2004.

McLeod, R.P. "Lumps, Bumps, Things That Go Itch in Yo Office!" *Journal of Schoo Nursing* 20(4):245-46, August 2004.

Middleton, C. "The Assessmen and Treatment of Patient with Chronic Pain," *Nurs Times* 100(18):40-44, May 2004.

Montgomery, R.K. "Pain Mana; ment in Burn Injury," *Critical Care Nursing Clinics of North Americ* 16(1):39-49, March 2004.

Potter, P.A. and Perry, A.G. *Fu damentals of Nursing*, 6 ed. St. Louis: Mosby–Yea Book, Inc., 2005.

Professional Guide to Signs a Symptoms, 4th ed. Philadelphia: Lippincott Willia & Wilkins, 2003.

en, R.L., Jr. "Neurologic
Assessment for Pronator
Drift," *Nursing2004*
34(3):22, March 2004.

*id Assessment: A Flowchart
Guide to Evaluating Signs
& Symptoms.* Philadelphia:
Lippincott Williams &
Wilkins, 2004.

*5 Portable RN: The All-in-One
Nursing Reference.* Phila-
delphia: Lippincott Williams
& Wilkins, 2005.

Walsh, S. "Formulation of a Plan
of Care for Culturally Di-
verse Patients," *International Journal of Nursing
Terminologies and Class-
ifications* 15(1):17-26,
January-March 2004.

Woodrow, P. "Assessing Blood
Pressure in Older People,"
Nursing Older People
16(1):29-31, March 2004.

Index

i refers to an illustration; t refers to a table.

i refers to an illustration; t refers to a table.

Throat pain, 120t, 122
Tics, 313
Transcultural communication, 46
Tremors, 306-307t, 313-314

U

Upper airway obstruction, signs and symptoms of, 143
Urethral meatus, displacement of, 246
Urinary frequency, urgency, and hesitancy, 216, 240, 243t
Urinary incontinence, 217, 219-220t, 244
Urine appearance, assessing, 228t
Urticaria, 72t, 74
Uterine prolapse, 223

V

Vaginal discharge, 220t
Vaginal prolapse, 223
Vaginitis, 221-222
Vascular system, assessing, 153-155, 156-157i, 157
Vertigo, 313
Vesicular rash, 74
Vision loss, 97
Visual acuity
  decreased, 93, 94-95t
  testing, 85-86, 87i
Visual floaters, 95t, 98
Visual halos, 98
Vital signs
  interpreting, 18
  measuring, 18-23
  recording, 18
Vocal fremitus, assessing, 137, 137i

WXYZ

Weber's test, 107, 108i
Weight
  body mass index and, 35
  categories of, 34
  excessive gain or loss in, 38-39
  measuring, 33-34
    in pediatric patient, 19
  as vital statistic, 18